Getting Your Best Health Care

Getting Your Best Health Care: Real-World Stories for Patient Empowerment

BY
KEN FARBSTEIN

PROFESSIONAL PATIENT ADVOCATE INSTITUTE
Washington, D.C.

© 2011 Access Intelligence, LLC, and Kenneth Farbstein.
All rights reserved. This publication may not be reproduced or transmitted in part or in full in any form or by any means, electronic or mechanical, including photocopying, recording and any information storage and retrieval system without first obtaining permission from the publisher.

Access Intelligence • 4 Choke Cherry Road, Second Floor • Rockville, MD 20850
www.accessintel.com
Professional Patient Advocate Institute • www.patientadvocatetraining.com
Dorland Health • www.dorlandhealth.com

In loving memory of Leo Juran

Table of Contents

INTRODUCTION 11

PART ONE: DURING A HEALTH CRISIS

    Chapter 1: Interacting with Your Doctor 17

    Chapter 2: Choosing Your Doctor 31

    Chapter 3: Choosing Surgery 47

    Chapter 4: Choosing Your Hospital and Surgeon 61

    Chapter 5: In the Hospital 67

    Chapter 6: In the Mental Health World 87

    Chapter 7: After the Error 99

    Chapter 8: Coping with Grave Illness 117

PART TWO: AT HOME

    Chapter 9: Coping with a Chronic Condition 127

    Chapter 10: Safe Complementary/Alternative Medicine 141

    Chapter 11: Living for Others 147

    Chapter 12: Finding and Working with a Professional Patient Advocate ... 155

    Chapter 13: Partners in the New Contract 167

APPENDIX: Favorites from Patient Safety Blog 173

> *"Each patient carries his own doctor inside him – we are at our best when we give the doctor who resides within each patient a chance to work."*
>
> —**Dr. Albert Schweitzer**

AUTHOR'S NOTE

All these stories are true, to the best of my knowledge. The true names of patients and their family members and friends appear here throughout this book, except where noted. In general, the names of their health care providers and those hospitals and medical groups associated with medical errors have been omitted. Those are identified only in exceptional cases, where their repeated errors have harmed a large number of people.

Introduction

William Halsted was a brilliant and famous doctor, but you wouldn't want him as your doctor. In 1882 he performed the first successful operation to remove gallstones. He performed the first emergency blood transfusion. He started the first formal surgical residency training program in the U.S., located at Johns Hopkins Hospital in Baltimore. He performed the first radical mastectomy for a patient with breast cancer.[1]

Yet he was addicted to cocaine and morphine. He refused to update his eyeglass prescription, leaving him with severely compromised vision. He was also forgetful, and sometimes kept patients waiting in the hospital for weeks at a time. None of them dared to ask him if it was time for him to perform their surgery.

Nowadays, our doctors can be just as smart as Dr. Halsted was. Few patients languish for weeks in the hospital while they await surgery. But patients are still way too timid, so other harms await us. How can we get the best care from our own very bright and yet all-too-human doctors and nurses? How to speak up to a brusque doctor?

The stories in this book teach us how to partner with our gifted doctors and nurses, to stay safe while in their care. Patients have relied for too long on the doctors' brilliance and goodness, believing that Doctor knows best. Doctors do know what's the best medical care, and we know what's best for us. It's time for us to step up as partners in our care.

I've come to realize that only in midlife, over the last few years. I've worked as an independent consultant, advising the doctors, nurses and administrators who lead hospitals and medical groups on improving the quality of care while limiting costs. My largest project was a three-year effort to help a multihospital system become the safest place in the world for a patient to get medication.

This culminated in 2001, when we won the largest award in hospital patient safety, the first Annual Premier Award in Hospital Medication Safety.

I had thought my future success in helping hospitals to improve medication safety, and patient safety more broadly, was assured. I marketed my services as aggressively as a good management consultant should. I was very surprised to find myself shunned. A good friend laughingly calls me an "anthrax salesman." Medical errors are a distasteful subject that no one in her right mind wants to be associated with. Hospital executives don't want outsiders to question their quality. And they certainly don't want to pay outsiders to do that; they believe they can improve quality on their own. In any event, there's no financial reason for them to improve quality: after errors occur, they get paid to meliorate them. I'm not saying they're evil; far from it. In the Boston suburb where I live, most of my close friends are doctors and nurses. They and their colleagues are good people who do the best they can in a system that sets up errors. Their bosses have a choice between buying a diagnostic machine that can generate revenue (or some other revenue-generating action), or hiring a consultant who won't generate revenue but might generate trouble. They'll take the revenue.

As I was learning this, a member of my family died from a medical error. At first the shock and grief paralyzed us. Later I realized I had to become far more vigilant, and far more active, in safeguarding the health of my family. I started noticing stories of medical error, and collecting them. I tried to use them in my consultation with hospitals, about as effectively as raising the volume of an anthrax salesman's sales pitch.

I had to do something. That's a key part of my Jewish faith: it's not enough to have a set of beliefs; one has to act on them to bring about social justice. I felt angry about the needless deaths and what it does to a victim's family members. I was scared about how the healthcare system might treat my father, ailing with Parkinson's disease. Many thousands of other people suffer and die needlessly each year, despite all the politically correct words about patient safety.

To empower patients, I started Patient Safety Blog (www.PatientSafetyBlog.com) in 2006. Most of the posts feature one person's story, with a suggestion for the patient on how to prevent a similar medical error from befalling them. This book adds significantly to the stories in the blog. A close friend, now a physician leader at Dana-Farber Cancer Institute, has a long-term dream of creating the new doctor. In my more lofty moments I think that this book might help create the new patient. And that we'll meet, like the construction of the first intercontinental railway, in the middle, together.

The stories in the first part of this book describe people's health crises. The first two chapters describe interactions with doctors, and choosing specialists and other doctors during a crisis. Following each story is a suggestion for patient advocates, whether they're professional advocates, family members or close friends. Such suggestions accompany the stories throughout the book. The third chapter discusses how people chose, and should choose, whether to have surgery. Chapters Four and Five describe how patients have chosen hospitals and surgeons, and stories of hospital care, respectively, with recommendations based on each story. Chapter Six offers stories of patients in the mental health world. Chapter Seven suggests what to do after a medical injury occurs, based on victims' experiences. Chapter Eight describes families' experiences with their decisions on treatment for grave illness.

The second part of the book describes the stories of people at home, living with chronic illness, and those who have sought alternative or complementary medicine, in Chapters Nine and Ten, respectively. Next is a set of stories about how some people have extended and improved their own lives through living for others. Chapter Twelve describes ways to find, choose, and work with professional patient advocates. The final chapter summarizes the emerging partnership between patients and their providers of care.

This book may find you in the midst of a health crisis. If so, you're already interacting with doctors and nurses, maybe even before you've consciously chosen them. We'll start there, with a story about a very widely known, and yet little known, celebrity.

Ken Farbstein
2011

---

1. Gerald Imber, Genius on the Edge: The Bizarre Double Life of Dr. William Sterwart Halsted, NY: Kaplan Publications, 2010.

PART ONE
During a Health Crisis

CHAPTER ONE

Interacting with Your Doctor

No matter what he did, he couldn't get to sleep. He had been sleeping poorly for quite a long time. So, in the middle of the night, he called the personal physician he had hired to get a sedative. It didn't work, so he called again, and got another sedative. He called a third time, getting a third sedative. Still frantic in the early morning, he called his doctor again and insisted on getting something that would knock him out. So finally his doctor gave him an injection that put him to sleep right away.

Within a few hours, this man, Michael Jackson, was pronounced dead.

The month before, in May 2009, Jackson had hired the physician, at $150,000 a month. That tragic night in June, the doctor had injected Jackson with Propofol, which apparently interacted with the tranquillizer Lorazepam that he had given Jackson earlier to help him sleep. The Lorazepam had slowed his breathing and heart rate, which the Propofol had slowed further, fatally, according to the coroner's report. The doctor also did not use the safeguards that constitute standard medical practice when Propofol is injected. No one had intubated Jackson's airway to ensure an ample inflow of oxygen, and no anesthesiologist was present, among other missing safeguards. Those errors may have been fatal, even if Lorazepam had not been used.[1]

What went wrong? Two root causes were working together. First, Jackson refused to be denied; he wouldn't take no for an answer from his doctor. In the police report, the doctor said he had finally relented, after trying for days to wean Michael off Propofol. Second, Jackson had chosen a doctor who flew solo. Normally a doctor would write a prescription; a pharmacist would review the prescription for safety before filling it, and the patient would take

> *"Helen's daughter and a friend testified that Helen could stay on the exercise machines for only a few minutes... She had been lying to Dr. Karr, playing the role of a good patient."*

the medicine. That process allows for a team of three to consider the medicine's safety: the doctor, the pharmacist, and the patient. Many retail pharmacists routinely use computers that immediately warn of any potentially dangerous interaction among drugs. For a drug like Propofol, which is usually used in hospitals during major surgery, the team would typically include an anesthesiologist and nurse as well. In this case, the doctor himself may have been groggy, like Jackson, so that neither of them could consider the right questions about the safe use of the drug. For the doctor to proceed then without a professional assistant, a cogent patient, or a computer was like a groggy pilot flying at night with no co-pilot or flight instrument panel: flying blind.

How could this have been prevented? With 20/20 hindsight, it's easy to say: The doctor should not have administered the injection as he did. He should not have let Jackson browbeat him. Jackson should have chosen a more professional and conscientious doctor and should have accepted the doctor's reluctance to order and provide Propofol. In the moment of a medical crisis, however, it's not so clear-cut. What should we do when we're in pain? Trust the doctor's judgment, and suffer? Or insist on prompt and effective treatment?

✚ Trust your doctor's judgment, and verify it. If the doctor says no, ask why. Keep an open mind, and explore safe treatment alternatives with your doctor.

Few patients have personal, live-in doctors who are always immediately available and willing to provide treatment, as Jackson did. Such a doctor is the one that most people think they want. But it's more important to have a doctor who can firmly and caringly say "no" and explain why; a doctor who uses nurses and other professional colleagues as backup, and who uses computer systems to warn of dangerous drug orders.

This book will use stories like this one to go beyond pat suggestions, and to identify ways you can partner with your doctor to get the best care. In cases like Jackson's, a judgment call was needed, precisely when his mind was most muddled. At times like that, it's useful to have a family member or professional as a patient advocate, to rely on their more objective judgment. The rest of this chapter discusses more tough judgment calls, organized by common issues between patients and doctors.

I DON'T WANT TO BOTHER THE DOCTOR

Stoic older men are known for not wanting to bother the doctor, though they need medical care. Others share the same tendency, as Keely's story shows:

> *A year ago, I ended up in the hospital with a severe kidney infection. I'd felt bad for a week, but I didn't want to bother the doctor with "just a bad backache" and some vague flu-y symptoms. I was training for a half-marathon and really busy with classes and I didn't want to deal with wasting my time on a doctor's visit over nothing. By the end of the week, I had a high fever and was in so much pain I could barely walk... and I was still telling myself it was probably just the flu and soreness from overtraining. I only got to the hospital when my boyfriend and roommate almost literally dragged me.*
>
> *I wouldn't feel so bad about it if it was just me affected by my delusional "it's nothing serious" thinking. But what followed that initial hospital admission was more than a week of worry for my family, a week of my boyfriend missing classes and work and sleeping in a hospital chair, and thousands of dollars worth of medical care.*[2]

➕ Older men, and all patients, need to change their image of strength from the uncomplaining tolerance of pain to endurance and survival over the longest time. To stay in the game and survive for the longest time, they'll sometimes need to get help from health care professionals. If you're in doubt, ask a friend or family member. That's especially important if you're macho, shy or elderly.

Sometimes people don't want to call the doctor because they don't think they're sick, or not sick enough. This can happen even with people who have significant diseases.

I WANT THE DOCTOR TO BE HAPPY WITH ME

Dr. Merilee Karr once treated a patient, "Helen Simmons," with chest pain.[3] Helen had gone to the emergency room of her local community hospital, and was admitted to the hospital overnight for observation. Dr. Karr examined her the next day. Blood tests revealed that she had not had a heart attack, though as a smoker with high blood pressure and a lengthy family history of heart disease, she was at high risk for one. Dr. Karr diagnosed heartburn.

Two weeks after she left the hospital, Simmons had a visit with Dr. Karr's partner. She reported that her pain was better, and a barium swallow (a special X-ray) showed that she had acid irritation of the stomach. Thinking she had heartburn, Dr. Karr's partner gave Simmons another prescription for an acid blocker.

Two weeks later, Simmons came to the clinic with bad chest pain, and Dr. Karr sent her to the hospital immediately for what turned out to be her first heart attack. In the hospital the cardiologists re-opened a heart artery.

Simmons joined a health club; she lost some weight and stayed off tobacco. Dr. Karr saw her every month or two over the next nine months, congratulating her each time for her progress.

She came in for a final visit that August, complaining of chest pain. An EKG showed nothing new; indeed, it showed some improvement. And Simmons reported that she was able to work out for hours without chest pain. Dr. Karr switched her to a stronger medicine for heartburn.

Ten days later, Simmons died of sudden cardiac death.

Her family brought a malpractice suit, claiming negligence. But Simmons' daughter and a friend testified that she could stay on the exercise machines for only a few minutes before she had to stop and rest until the chest pain went away. She had been lying to Dr. Karr, playing the role of a good patient.

Dr. Karr was found not guilty, but she feels responsible for not seeing through her patient's performance.

> ✚ Always tell the doctor the truth, even if it's uncomfortable. The doctor will feel more proud of you – and of herself, if there's a genuine cure – than if you pretend that everything is fine. If it's awkward to tell your doctor something, ask a friend or relative to talk to the doctor.

I'M WORRIED THAT OUT OF FRIENDSHIP MY DOCTOR MIGHT TREAT ME WITH KID GLOVES

Beyond wanting to be a good patient, people often feel quite friendly with their doctor. That's fine, usually, but if the doctor considers himself more of a friend than a doctor, he may be reluctant to cause some necessary discomfort. So an elderly man with thyroid cancer told a friendly doctor, "Don't save me from an unfriendly test just because we're friends." That enabled his doctor, an endocrinologist [who treats disorders of the body's hormone production systems] at a large urban teaching hospital, to recommend a difficult treatment regimen involving radioactive iodine. Out of her friendship with the man, she had been reluctant to provide that treatment, as it was likely to greatly disrupt his life.[4]

> Dr. Jerome Groopman suggests that in such situations you can say to the doctor, "You should know how deeply I appreciate how much care you show. Please know also that I understand you may need to do things that cause discomfort or pain."

ONLY SICK PEOPLE TAKE DRUGS, AND I DON'T WANT TO BE A SICK PERSON

Dr. Dena Rifkin once treated a man who had waited for many years for a kidney transplant. He had been undergoing four-hour dialysis sessions for years. A kidney finally became available, and the transplant operation went well. Her patient faithfully took the immunosuppressive medicine (to keep his body from rejecting the new kidney) twice a day for 10 months, with no side effects, and he was able to eat and drink whatever he wanted.

Then her patient accidentally missed a dose – and he noticed that nothing happened. Then he went away for a week, deliberately not taking his medicine, again with no perceptible harm.

Within two months, however, his body started rejecting the new kidney. Now the kidney was barely functioning, landing him in the hospital again.

He had thought he was healthy – and that healthy people didn't need dialysis, and didn't need to take medicine.[6]

> ✚ If you'd like to reduce or stop taking your prescribed medication, let your doctor know that, and discuss it. That's especially important if you're on strong medication, or if you've been hospitalized for a related condition. You can call and leave a message. Better yet, if the doctor uses email, send an email message to the doctor, so you'll be able to refer back later to his email reply to remind you of the dosage decision the two of you reached and the reasons for it.

MY KID IS SCARED TO GO TO THE DOCTOR

Sometimes children need to sit still during a difficult medical procedure or treatment. Medical play therapists have developed ways to work with young cancer patients. Their techniques can be useful for other children too. Dr. Cori Liptak of Dana-Farber Cancer Institute in Boston helps prepare children for cancer treatment ahead of time, so they understand what their job will be. She'll engage in medical play with a child, having the child, for example, give shots to a puppet. They'll tell the puppet, "We'll put on your magic cream now, so it will numb the spot, and you won't feel a thing. Don't be scared." Or she'll have the child pretend to sit like a statue.[7]

> ✚ Mothers, you can engage in this kind of play with your child before a medical appointment if your child fears the doctor. Knowledge, and laughter, are the enemies of fear.

MY KID'S MEDS AREN'T WORKING. WHAT DO I DO?

Suzanne Joblonski wrote in the *New York Times*:

> *I am the mother of a teenage boy who received a diagnosis of attention deficit disorder and oppositional defiant disorder eight years ago and was prescribed antipsychotic medication. Throughout the years, we have visited no fewer than five psychiatrists and countless other therapists.*

I would often question why my son was prescribed medications (at one point three at a time) that failed to do as they promised. For example, the ones that were designed to help him sleep at night did the reverse, and the ones [prescribed] to keep him awake made him lethargic.

I decided that it was in my son's best interest to take a break from the weekly therapy and daily medication. Surprisingly, he functioned much better. His sleeping patterns and appetite improved. He is now back on medication, but with new therapists and with the parents' considerations in mind.

Families like ours are often duped into believing that there aren't options other than medication, or [that] should we refuse to comply, charges of neglect could be brought.[8]

✚ If your child's medications don't have the desired effects, talk to your doctor and your family about your alternatives. After that, make a conscious decision, like Suzanne did.

SHOULD I BRING MY SICK CHILD TO THE PEDIATRICIAN?

As a father with 20 years of parenting experience, I sometimes have to decide whether to bring my child to the pediatrician. If it will help, of course, I'll bring in my son or daughter, but if not, I'd rather not spend the time. So I call the doctor's office and talk to either the receptionist or the nurse, and decide with them whether my kid's complaint is worth a doctor's visit. It's helpful to have guidance ahead of time from the doctor's office.

Some pediatricians are starting to think more systematically about how to partner with their patients in making this decision. Dr. Lester Hartman of Westwood-Mansfield Pediatrics outside of Boston has been particularly innovative in several ways.

In Dr. Hartman's office, staff routinely collect the email addresses of their young patients' parents. He sends an e-newsletter to teach the parents when to come in for a sore throat, what croup looks like, and so forth. He says:

> *One Saturday while I was on call, the nurse practitioner and I must have seen 30 children with influenza. It was the same old story: the child has a cough and complains of a sore throat and achiness. The parent focuses on the sore throat, worrying about strep or pneumonia. We sent out an e-mail that evening telling parents: "We often realize that when parents bring their child into the office during flu season, they are often concerned about pneumonia or strep throat. Interestingly, most children who complain of sore throats say it is a minor symptom compared to their headaches and body aches. If your child says this when you ask then it is unlikely to be strep. Coughs and high fevers are very common in flu season and do not represent pneumonias. Call if your child has the following symptoms...Remember your child can have a fever for five to seven full days." The next day we saw two-thirds fewer children with the flu.*

In this way Dr. Hartman was able to tell most of the parents – i.e., the vast majority who had email – what to watch for, and how to respond.[9]

➕ Get a pediatrician like Dr. Hartman.

I'M WORRIED THAT A PRESCRIBED DRUG MIGHT HAVE BAD SIDE EFFECTS

Robert Jones woke up at 3 a.m. one day with a big toe the size of a sausage. It was so painful, he said, that he couldn't keep a blanket on. He made an appointment to see a rheumatologist (a doctor specializing in joints, and in soft and connective tissue) at New England Baptist Hospital in Boston. The doctor there prescribed two drugs for gout. Robert looked into them and read about their possible side effects. Concerned, he didn't fill the prescriptions.

Not long afterward, while in Italy, he had a terrible gout attack that affected his ankle, knees and feet, and came home in a wheelchair. He went back to the doctor and now takes a combination of drugs. He's doing well. His doctor woke him up, he says, adding: "I don't need to suffer unnecessarily."[10]

➕ If you're concerned about the possible side effects of medicine your doctor has prescribed, ask your doctor and your pharmacist how to minimize the side effects while getting the most benefit from the drugs. They might suggest, for example, changing the frequency with which you take the drugs, or an extended-release form of the drug.

I'M WORRIED THAT MY DOCTOR MIGHT BE SKIPPING SOME IMPORTANT TESTS

You might expect that your doctor will perform certain tests and be surprised and even disappointed if he doesn't do so. Dr. Gabriel Ledger explains a doctor's mind-set in this letter to the *New Yorker*:

> *A major impediment to minimizing patient testing is patient expectation. My patient with a viral chest cold expects a chest X-ray to prove that his two-week cough isn't pneumonia (it isn't), and the mother of my 3-year-old patient who tumbled off the sofa expects a CT scan to prove that everything will be fine with the child's brain (it will be fine, except for the unknown long-term results of the radiation from the CT scan). When the tests aren't done, the patients leave my E.R. dissatisfied and write complaint letters to the hospital. And, in the rare instance that the viral chest cold later turns into pneumonia, the patient assumes that I "missed it" and wants to sue me. Doctors need to be held accountable for over-testing, but let's not forget how patient expectation affects the issue.[11]*

➕ If you expect a test to be done and it's not ordered, say something like, "I thought we'd need a test for that. Isn't that necessary? Can you explain that, please?"

I'M SURPRISED THAT THAT'S WHAT THE DOCTOR THINKS IS MY DIAGNOSIS

Sometimes one suspects, or a close friend suspects, that a diagnosis is wrong. According to her boyfriend, the Brazilian model Mariana Bridi da Costa initially was told by her doctor that she had kidney stones, which occur very rarely in young women. The doctor prescribed medication for the kidney stones and sent her home. Da Costa was later found to have actually had a severe urinary tract infection, which worsened, bringing her back to the hospital two days later. The infection spread to her blood (septicemia), which led to major organ failure and her death.[12]

➕ If you doubt the diagnosis, ask the doctor what else it might be.

Donna Pikula offers an example of what to do when you doubt a diagnosis. She spent months being treated for acid-reflux-like symptoms, seeing doctor after doctor. Acid reflux is a common problem, in which stomach acid flows backward from the stomach up to the esophagus. Donna had a history of thyroid conditions in her family, which made her think that her problem might be related to her thyroid gland. Indeed, she asked specifically whether her symptoms might be caused by a thyroid condition. But her doctors brushed her off, telling her to keep taking the "little purple pill."

The diagnosis of acid reflux didn't make sense to Donna because she had always been able to eat whatever she wanted without any problems, and yet now even eating cereal or drinking water was painful.

After undergoing many tests ordered by various specialists, Donna finally referred herself to an endocrinologist – a specialist in thyroid diseases – at a large medical center. He was immediately certain that her symptoms were due to her body's production of too much thyroid hormone (hyperthyroidism). Testing confirmed his diagnosis. Donna had surgery to remove her thyroid gland, and now takes daily thyroid hormone replacement.[13]

"The patient's religious faith forbade any blood transfusions, even from his own blood."

➕ Be persistent in seeking a diagnosis that makes sense to you. Find a specialist in another field with expertise in the condition you suspect you have. If you're not sure of the appropriate specialty, ask a friend who's a nurse or doctor.

MY DOCTOR HAS DIFFERENT VALUES AND ASSUMPTIONS THAN I DO, WHICH MIGHT LEAD HER TO GIVE ME INAPPROPRIATE OR UNACCEPTABLE TREATMENT

Surgeon Bruce Campbell once saw a patient who was a Jehovah's Witness. The man needed him to remove a large noncancerous goiter (a swelling in the thyroid gland) in his upper chest.

The patient's religious faith forbade any blood transfusions, even from his own blood. In the initial office visit, he informed Dr. Campbell about his convictions serenely and matter-of-factly. He was clearly aware that serious consequences could occur if there was bleeding during the operation (which would normally require a transfusion). Dr. Campbell reluctantly agreed to perform the operation on those terms.

More anxious than his patient, he performed the surgery – successfully.[14]

> ✚ Calmly and clearly discuss with your doctor any relevant religious or spiritual specifications for your treatment beforehand. It's helpful if you can learn about the key trade-offs and possible consequences before that conversation.

Another occasion when there is often a gap between what a patient expects and what a doctor assumes occurs at the end of life. Doctors are trained to fight disease and to do all they can to extend life, but some patients prefer them not to act so aggressively to extend life. This is discussed further in Chapter 8.

MY DOCTOR IS SO BUSY WITH TECHNOLOGY I WORRY THAT HE WON'T LISTEN TO ME

Some doctors would like to listen better than they do. A stethoscope amplifies very quiet heart and lung sounds, but if the patient speaks that sends a painfully loud blast of noise into both the doctor's ears. On one such occasion 30 years ago, Dr. Richard Baron snapped to his talking patient, "Shhh. I can't hear you while I'm listening." He heard himself, stopped, and laughed, realizing the irony of his statement, and wrote a classic article on the topic.[15]

That's the key challenge facing doctors in modern medical practice: to listen and perceive with all senses and with all available technology – while remembering to listen to the patient's voice.

For a patient who typically has a limited time with the doctor, it's hard to achieve the right balance of letting the doctor do her thing while telling her what she needs to know.

> ✚ Because your time with the doctor is so limited, you'll need to be prepared, so bring a list of your key questions, and send them to the doctor in advance. Bring a printed list to the appointment. If your problem is complicated, you can even bring a typed paragraph summarizing it, which should save time during the appointment.

I WANT SOME CONTROL OVER MY TREATMENT AT TIMES WHEN I FEEL SO WEAK AND POWERLESS

Doctors can sometimes schedule drug regimens of chemotherapy or steroids around major events like birthday parties. One patient, described by cancer doctor Holcombe Grier, worked with his doctor to rearrange a chemo treatment around an upcoming Bruce Springsteen concert.

Dr. Grier, who works with young patients, says, "At almost any age, there is a desire to exert some control over your environment. Medical residents need to be thoughtful in doing rounds with me and ask a child, 'I have to listen to your chest. Do you want me to do it here, or do you want to stand over there by Mommy?'"[16]

> ✚ Talk to your doctor about ways to fit your medical treatment into your life, so that it doesn't substitute for it. Keep doing the things that make life worth living for you, like Springsteen concerts.

I WANT MY CARE TO BE TAILORED TO MY PERSONAL NEEDS

As my friend Dr. Saul Weingart says, "We all want a tailor, but it's an off-the-rack world." I second that emotion. To get individualized attention during my own physical exam, I email my primary care physician a list of my questions, in descending order of importance, a couple of days before the appointment. The day before the appointment, I fax a copy of the list to his office, requesting that they give it to him early the next morning. I bring a copy to the appointment, and he answers my questions when he's ready to. The advance copies let him think about his answers ahead of time, and allow time to refresh his medical knowledge about my own issues as needed.

✚ Let your doctor know your concerns in writing before your office visit.

I'M GRATEFUL TO MY DOCTOR

Blogger Christine Miserandino has frequent doctor's appointments for her lupus. She knows how busy the doctor is, and respects his time.

She fosters a relationship with her doctor, as she knows that her health greatly depends on him. "I do care," she says, "because I want him to care about me. I bring cookies at Christmastime. It's a relationship you have to foster like any other." Once, after a doctor visited her twice in the hospital in one day, she wrote a thank-you note – the first he had received in 20 years.[5]

After my own screening colonoscopy – one's 50th birthday present, the staff call that – I was able to write a one-word thank-you note to the doctor in his native Portuguese, using my entire knowledge of the language and all of my mental acuity during the conscious sedation. He was so touched that he wrote a you're welcome letter. In English.

✚ Thank your doctor in a way that will be meaningful to her. You are in a relationship, where thoughtfulness will go a long way.

YOUR PROFESSIONAL PATIENT ADVOCATE CAN:

Before the visit:

- Allay some of your fears about seeing the doctor.
- Prepare a list of questions for you to discuss with your doctor, and transmit the list to the doctor.

During the visit:

- Accompany you to the doctor's office, record the conversation, and translate the doctor's language into terms you'll understand.

Between visits:

- Set up a system reminding you to take your medicine.

- Look into alternatives to your medications to consider with your doctor.

- Check for drug-drug interactions.

- Look into the value of certain diagnostic tests for people with your condition, for discussion with your doctor.

- Suggest other diagnoses for consideration by your doctor, if you doubt your diagnosis.

- Give you information so you feel more empowered at a vulnerable time.

---

1. Coroner's Report, Case Number 2009-04415, at www.thesmokinggun.com/archive/years/2010/0208101jackson17.html. James McKinley, Jr., "Differing Sides of Physician who Tended to Jackson," New York Times, September 26, 2009.
2. Keely [sic], "Connection Disconnection" blog, August 9, 2010, at http://disconnectedgeek.wordpress.com/2010/08/09/i-am-a-monster/
3. Merilee Karr, "Missing," In: Silence Kills: Speaking Out and Saving Lives, Creative Nonfiction, Issue #33, 2007.
4. Jerome Groopman, How Doctors Think, New York: Mariner Books, 2007, pages 54-55; 58.
5. Elizabeth Cohen and Jennifer Pifer, "Are You an Obnoxious Patient?", CNN, January 24, 2008 at www.wibw.com/home/headlnes/14181067.html
6. Dena Rifkin, "A Holiday from Illness, All too Fleeting," New York Times, April 22, 2008, page D6.
7. Cori Liptak (edited by Dawn Stapleton), First Person, Paths of Progress, published by Dana-Farber Cancer Institute, Fall/Winter 2008, page 31.
8. Suzanne Joblonski, "Giving Psychiatric Drugs to Children," New York Times, Letters to the Editor, December 16, 2009, page A36.
9. Interviews with Lester Hartman, July 2009. See also www.WMPeds.com
10. Laura Duffy, "Innovations at New England Baptist Hospital," Summer 2009.
11. Gabriel Ledger, New Yorker, June 29, 2009, letter to the editor.
12. Shari Roan, "Beauty queen's amputation is rare complication of septicemia," Los Angeles Times, January 23, 2009, at http://latimesblogs.latimes.com/booster_shots/2009/01/beauty-queens-a.html
13. Donna Pikula, After the Diagnosis: How to Look Out for Yourself or a Loved One, Hartland, MI: Books to Help You, 2006, pages xv-xvi.
14. Bruce Campbell, "Listening to Leviticus," JAMA, February 27, 2008, pages 879-80.
15. Abigail Zuger, "The Tools of Doctors, and a Price for Patients," New York Times, October 27, 2009.
16. Saul Wisnia, "Ups and Downs: Taking the Steps to Recovery," Paths of Progress, Fall/Winter 2008, pages 14-15.

CHAPTER TWO

Choosing Your Doctor

It's magical and compelling. A patient experiences a rare and inexplicable set of symptoms, and yet within the hour, less time for the commercials, the quirky Dr. House is always able to diagnose and successfully treat the condition.

How to find the real-life doctors like the ones on TV? They really exist, though they usually live far from Hollywood. Real-life Hollywood doctors can be too star-struck to provide high-quality care. Indeed, Michael Jackson's doctor has been the subject of a criminal investigation.[1]

The psychiatrist for another celebrity, a former model and sex symbol, is also involved in a criminal investigation about the reasons for a patient's death. Anna Nicole Smith's psychiatrist testified that a month after her death, the psychiatrist had gathered 44 different prescription drugs from Anna's seaside home and brought them to the county office of the chief toxicologist. The drugs had had fatal interactive effects: the autopsy report identified the combination of choral hydrate, a sedative/sleeping agent, with benzodiazepines (anti-anxiety/anti-depressive medicine) and Benadryl as the mechanism of her death. Multiple injections of "longevity drugs" in her buttocks had caused viral enteritis – deep tissue abscesses. That, and the flu, also contributed to her death.[2]

Doctors for both Michael and Anna appear to have pandered to their celebrity patients, and to have communicated and collaborated inadequately with other doctors. They showed poor judgment. They apparently didn't use computer systems that would automatically warn of dangerous drug interactions. This chapter discusses the use of databases of physicians to select a doctor. In light of the databases' limitations, the issues in finding Dr. Right, who has

> *"A study of more than 1 million patients' doctors concluded that these publicly available characteristics are poor proxies for ascertaining doctors' likely performance. "*

31

generous empathy, objectivity and deep technical skill, and appropriate supplemental office systems in a single human being, are discussed in turn.

USING DATABASES

How to find the best doctor for you? Many people nowadays find a doctor via a list of the best doctors, or look online at databases. But beware: most aren't based on evidence about the health outcomes of the doctors' patients. Instead, many of them rely on characteristics of doctors like their education, certification by a board, and malpractice history. A study of more than 1 million patients' doctors, published in the *Archives of Internal Medicine*, concluded that these publicly available characteristics are poor proxies for ascertaining doctors' likely performance on clinical quality measures. That said, three characteristics were associated with overall performance, though the link was very slight: female gender, board certification, and graduation from a medical school in the U.S.[3]

Some lists of best doctors may be influenced by a magazine's hopes for advertising revenue. One list is produced by Key Professional Media, which makes a business of creating these "super" lists for various geographic areas. Its website calls the advertising opportunities "a great way to reach a wealth of new patients and referral sources [and] helps brand you as one of the leading physicians in your area." Apparently, Key basically buys a section of a magazine, labels it a "special advertising section," and sells the advertising space to doctors. One of the "super doctors" in the "Texas Super Doctors 2005" list had lost the biggest malpractice suit in the county's history, for $600 million, and a month later, another patient under his care died from a chemotherapy overdose. While it's conceivable that a doctor with two such tragedies might still be a "super doctor," the errors should have been mentioned on his listing. The Super Doctors website admits in its fine print that "selecting a physician is an important decision that should not be based solely on advertising or listings in this website."[4] Indeed!

For *D Magazine* in the Dallas area, doctors vote, and then a panel of doctors selects the "best" ones. This process identified 572 doctors as Dallas' "Best Doctors" in 2005, 643 in 2006, 611 in 2007, 678 in 2008, and 729 in 2009.[5]

✚ In choosing a doctor, get the help of a professional patient advocate. Or use a web site that rates the report cards: http://InformedPatientInstitute.org can steer you toward an appropriate, highly rated report card website that identifies the best physicians in your own state.

Perhaps the most renowned name in consumer ratings is *Consumer Reports*, published by Consumers Union. In September 2010, CU began making available to subscribers its rankings of surgeons who perform coronary artery bypass grafts (CABGs).[6] The ratings only describe each surgeon's medical group as average, above average, or below average – and only a very small minority are identified as "below average." Apparently most of the groups that would have been considered "below average" chose to withhold permission for Consumers Union to make their ratings public. Still, these ratings do mark an early milestone, and are somewhat useful.

Of course, most people don't pick a doctor by looking in a database. People with serious illnesses often rely on the suggestion of another doctor. That worked quite well for former vice presidential candidate Geraldine Ferraro. Feeling chronically tired after her U.S. Senate campaign in 1998, she learned at her annual checkup that she had either leukemia, lymphoma, or multiple myeloma. Her internist sent her to a cancer doctor (an oncologist/hematologist), who suggested a particular specialist in multiple myeloma. He has directed her care since then, and 12 years later, now at age 75, she has greatly outlived her initial prognosis of three to five years.[7]

EMPATHY IN USE

I still remember my father's belly laugh, long ago, when he heard of the possibility that computers could suggest diagnoses, and could even one day replace doctors. The idea that an automaton could substitute for a wise and warm confidante was ridiculous. Father knew best, as the following story shows.

Patients are often fearful when they see a doctor, worrying about what is really wrong with them, and how serious it is. That was certainly true for Cynthia, a well-dressed middle-aged woman who came to a new dentist, Dr. George Reskakis, complaining of bad breath, and wanting a teeth cleaning. As part of his standard conversation with a new patient, he explained the need for a proper evaluation, including X-rays. She unequivocally refused. He explained the rationale for them, and then discussed the guidelines of the American Dental Association, the modern, digital system of X-rays, and the quickness and painlessness of the minimal radiation she'd receive. The conversation itself took 15 minutes. Finally, she reluctantly agreed. She needed quite a bit of work: root canals, gum surgery, two posts and two crowns. Only afterward did she confide the reason she had resisted so stubbornly: her mother had died from cancer due to radiation treatment as a child. So they talked again about radiation and the vastly lower doses used nowadays.

As Dr. Reskakis explains,

> *...in a profession where anxiety is often the starting point of a doctor-patient relationship, the standard patient questionnaire will never go deep enough. Asking about flossing habits won't lead to fears that trace to events 60 years ago. In our armchair-psychology way, we hope to get to that level of trust eventually. In the meantime, we clean and drill, and insist on X-rays.*[8]

✚ In considering diagnostic tests, find a doctor who will listen to your concerns and take the time to discuss them with you.

"Anne Dodge" eventually found such a doctor, after meeting perhaps 30 doctors during her 15-year bout of a mysterious illness. None of Anne's four sisters had a similar illness. Around age 20, she found that food did not agree with her. She had no appetite, and when she forced herself to eat she'd feel sick and would regurgitate it. She had a series of infections. Deteriorating, she was hospitalized four times in 2004 to try to gain weight under supervision, without success. Her internist and psychiatrist thought she was not telling the truth about her steady weight loss.

Finally she saw a stomach doctor (a gastroenterologist), who asked her to tell her story from the start, without interruption. He began with a general, open-ended question about when she had begun to feel ill, many years before. He sensed that she felt emotions that blocked her from telling the story. So he made sure to respond sympathetically as she spoke. The detail of her story, his examination, and tests enabled Dr. Myron Falchuk to arrive at the diagnosis of an allergy to gluten (present in many grains), which is called celiac sprue, an autoimmune disorder. Able to adjust her diet accordingly, Anne gained 12 pounds in the next month. The doctor's active listening to the information she provided had saved her.[9]

Together, he and she had produced the diagnosis. That's particularly important for patients who have long been struggling with conditions that are difficult to diagnose and to treat. Dr. Stephen Bergman offers another example:

> *Decades ago when I was a medical student in Boston at one of man's greatest hospitals, I was assigned a woman with "difficulty breathing." She was 56 years old, a mother of three whose husband had died two years before. In good health all her life, she worked in a flower shop. She had never before had trouble breathing. Her husband's death had been a shock, but with the support of friends and family she had gotten through it pretty well. The resident – my boss – came in and took her history, in a rat-a-tat technique of asking a probing question that had to be answered yes or no, and as soon as there was a response, cutting her off and moving on to the next. I knew he was filling in his grid, a decision tree that would provide the diagnosis. No new information came up. A physical exam showed nothing but her panting. Lab work revealed increased eosinophilia, the blood cell that increases when the body is allergic to something. The resident went back and grilled her on allergies. Nothing.*
>
> *Her workup proceeded in classic academic fashion, with increasingly refined blood tests and X-rays. The latter showed a diffuse pattern of lung irritation, but no lesions or tumors. Experts were called in, and each diagnosed something in their area of expertise, from the psychiatrist diagnosing "melancholia" at her husband's death, to the surgeons wanting to cut. She kept getting worse, the oxygen levels in her blood falling lower and lower, bluing her lips, paling her face. A look of doom seemed to cloud her eyes. The surgeons did a lung biopsy, which showed only that her lung was reacting to some antigen, as the blood test had shown.*
>
> *She continued to decline. Palliative treatment was begun. The resident and staff doctors seemed reluctant to enter her room. I felt scared*

for her and sorry, and spent more and more time sitting with her, just talking – a medical student has time for this arcane procedure. One day I asked her where she lived. She said that after her husband died she'd taken in boarders to survive. I asked about them. "One of them's... a real trip," she gasped. "A magician." I smiled and asked more about him. Part of his act involved trained pigeons, which he kept in cages in the basement. "The cages are right above my washer/dryer." My ears perked up. It turned out that whenever she ran the dryer, the pigeon droppings were aerosolized and she breathed them in – for the past two years. I rushed to the medical library – in those days we still used books – and found "Pigeon Breeder's Lung Disease." Treatment: get rid of the pigeons; and a course of steroids. Prognosis: excellent. The magician suffered. She got well.

If we rely on technology and tests and neglect "being with" the patient, we may well miss the vital human facts that will solve the mystery and bring the cure.[10]

Dr. Bergman found the time to be with the patient. It's not clear whether he had explicitly asked her to help him play detective. A few years ago, when I saw a dermatologist for a sudden rash that looked like a bad case of acne, she said we'd need to play detective, to think about what recent changes might have caused this. Later, at home, I realized that I had bought and used a different brand of shaving cream. I brought it in, together with a can of my usual brand. She compared the ingredients, and identified Red Dye #20 as the likely culprit. I've read the fine print ever since, and have never had a recurrence of the rash.

In such "co-production of a diagnosis," it's important for the patient to discuss the timing of symptoms with the doctor. Dr. Bernard Lown discussed the case of a college president who had a very serious heart rhythm disorder (ventricular tachycardia) for more than 10 years. When asked, the patient told Dr. Lown that the arrhythmia occurred consistently in the morning, between 7:30 and 8:30 a.m. Dr. Lown realized that the man's medication had been wearing off by early morning. The man was taking an overly large dose at intervals around the clock, provoking many adverse symptoms without containing the arrhythmia. Instead, Dr. Lown told him to wake up and take a double dose at 5:30 a.m., and go back to sleep. By doing this for the next eight years, the patient had a normal heart rhythm.[11]

✚ Keep notes on the timing of your symptoms, and share that with your doctor.

Certain kinds of questions, answers and discussions are important in treatment of chronic conditions, not only in their diagnosis, as in this story of "Patty," a friend of mine:

> *When I was 14, I suffered from a series of unexplained seizures, and ever since then, debilitating migraine headaches. It is said that the function of the human brain is one of medicine's last remaining mysteries. I believe that the function (or should I say dysfunction?) of our health care system is equally confounding. When I first moved to Boston after college, my seizures and headaches were well controlled.*
>
> *Soon after I started my first job, I was stricken by an intractable migraine. I was newly endowed with health insurance, so I picked a doctor's name out of a directory. I was 22, and it seemed as good a method as any for choosing a PCP. My doctor asked me briskly why I'd come, and I explained about the relentless headache and my complex neurological history. I requested a referral to a neurologist. "I don't think you need to see a neurologist," she said dismissively. "I want you to try taking Sudafed – " she scribbled the dosage on a pad – "and see if that helps." I knew my condition – and my suffering – was far beyond the powers of Sudafed, and I tried to convey that. But the doctor smiled tightly, gathered up her papers, and left the room. When the Sudafed failed, my PCP informed me that no in-network neurologist could see me before March, which, after all, "was only two months away".*
>
> *After days of diligent effort and calls to three different hospitals, I finally wrangled an earlier appointment. By then I was enraged. The pain had become excruciating, and so had the indignity of having to negotiate the privilege of medical care. I recounted the whole saga to the neurologist. He nodded thoughtfully, stroking his beard and taking notes. I hoped he was jotting down ideas for fast-tracking my future appointments. Finally, he asked how I was feeling. I sighed, trembling now. "I feel horrible. I'm really hoping you can give me something for the pain." The physician paused and then his face closed. "I don't think I can work with you if you're going to be so demanding. I'm going to refer*

you to another neurologist; hopefully he can accommodate you better." I nodded politely, deeply humiliated. I thought about the rain outside, the missed morning of work, all the effort wasted for this referral, for which I'd lobbied so hard. I believe that it was only through family connections that I gained access to a headache specialist who ended my misery and prescribed medication that has helped me for years.

But sadly, the story doesn't end there. After several years of equilibrium, the intensive stress of graduate school wreaked further havoc on my system. I met with yet another provider, who prescribed a medication that I knew lowers seizure threshold. In fact, I said, I had taken the same medication as a teenager, right before I experienced my first seizure. The doctor was cavalier. "Those seizures were almost 20 years ago; I think you'll be fine." Without consulting any member of my health care team or reviewing my medical records, he wrote me a prescription. Then he left for vacation.

Exactly two weeks later, a grand mal seizure rendered me unconscious. I fell down on the sidewalk and woke up in an ambulance. Completely disoriented, I barely knew where – or who – I was. I spent the night in the hospital, and then began the process anew. Finding specialists. Begging for appointments. Demanding coverage from the stingy grad school health insurance. Eventually stabilizing the situation with different medications (expensive drugs that I will have to take for the foreseeable future) and caring providers.

I remain stunned that I received such uneven care in a city renowned for its medical resources. I've learned that the best providers are the most difficult to access, and that our flawed and complicated health care system often undermines the best intentions of health care and insurance providers. Through my experiences, I've learned to advocate for myself and my health.

Three different doctors came up short in empathy, in different ways. Patty's primary care physician had devalued Patty's eight years of knowledge about her disease, in denying her access to a neurologist and in prescribing Sudafed. When Patty described her excruciating pain, the first neurologist called her "so demanding" for asking for pain medicine. The final provider prescribed a drug that lowers the seizure threshold, and indeed, had shortly preceded a seizure she'd had years before. He prescribed it despite her explicit statement about that, neither consulting anyone in her health care team nor reviewing her medical records.[12]

Patty was an experienced patient who knew how the system works. Patients who are themselves nurses or doctors are also often acutely aware of their own doctors' limitations, as nurse practitioner Richard Ferri describes:

> *I am so damn tired of this...I am not my T cell count or viral load level and I wish to hell people would stop treating me like I am. It is degrading, and worse yet, it puts up roadblocks to communication between friends, medical providers, and the rest of the damn world.*
>
> *I have been practicing AIDS medicine since the beginning of the epidemic. Today is very different and as a clinician I am a much happier man because of the advances in HIV therapy. But we have become a community that is still fixated on clinical numbers and not the person sitting in front of us and this had got to stop.*
>
> *I recently felt compelled to change my AIDS doc because all I was was just a bunch of numbers to her. I was the "good" patient. She knew I took care of myself, was sober, worked out, and was nearly perfect with sticking to my meds. So I got the "greet them, treat them and street them" kind of medical care all clinicians fall into now and then on a regular basis. So after numerous attempts of talking with her about my care concerns and not seeing things change I said the short version of the Serenity Prayer, which is "F--- it!", and found another provider who is wonderful. She treats me like a real person. I am a real person! She asks what is going on in my life and my numbers, while still important, are not the heart and soul of every visit.*
>
> *I have had several other medical conditions overlooked because of my being a "good patient" that I had to handle myself. But I am lucky because I am an AIDS-certified nurse practitioner and knew how to get the help I needed. What about the average person with HIV/AIDS without that sort of background? What happens to them? I assume they fall through the clinical cracks and suffer.*[13]

Richard was able to find a doctor who treats him like a real person. He knew he didn't have to settle for a doctor who saw him only as a series of numbers, and acted on that knowledge. When nurses and doctors become patients, they often act as empowered patients. It's important for laymen to act that way, though it may feel less natural.

It can be especially difficult to find an empathic doctor when a language barrier blocks easy communication by the patient. Sometimes a medical interpreter can help as a negotiator, or even a problem-solver. One afternoon in September 2008 in Hennepin County Medical Center in Minneapolis, doctors decided that they needed to draw blood for a test to determine what ailed a Somali patient. The patient refused, thinking it would be a sin to draw blood at that time, which was during the holy month of Ramadan. The interpreter and doctor negotiated with the patient, finally calling an imam. The Muslim spiritual leader declared there was no sin, and the patient's blood was drawn. Here, both the patient and the doctor had made known their concerns, and both were open-minded in listening to an outside authority.[14]

"If you feel pressured to participate in a clinical trial of a new drug, you can ask who makes it, and later ask the office manager in confidence if the doctor gets money from that company."

Sometimes doctors think they're being engaging, and defusing anxiety, when they're not. Here's a nurse's letter to an advice columnist:

> *"Dr. Sam," a good-natured general surgeon in our same-day surgery clinic, enjoys chatting with patients before procedures. To put them at ease, he regales them with humorous stories, and most of them love it. Last week, Dr. Sam told several of his favorite stories to a patient who was clearly anxious. After he left, she confided to me that she was still dreading surgery. "I had some questions that I never got to ask because he was too busy being a comedian," she said.*[15]

It's tough to be a doctor nowadays. Most of the patients love the doctor's humor, which eases their anxiety. Though laughter may be the best medicine, it doesn't work for everyone. You're entitled to request that your care be tailored to you.

➕ If your doctor is too chatty, get a list of your questions to the office manager or nurse ahead of time, noting your concern about whether the doctor will have time to answer them.

OBJECTIVITY

You'll be able to sense the doctor's empathy, or lack of it. It will be harder to sense her objectivity. You'd like to think your doctor is objective, and not influenced by conflicts of interest. Maybe. Drug companies often pay for very nice trips for doctors to exotic locations, and pay nicely for doctors' lectures to other doctors about their drugs. A physician friend – a well-regarded doctor – recently mentioned he had been a "Pfizer prostitute" by accepting an honorarium to give a talk to his fellow physician specialists, using slides prepared by the drug maker. Doctors who do that aren't evil; as my friend explained, someone else would do it, if he didn't, and he has a kid in college to pay for. But he can't be fully objective anymore.

A surprising number of doctors, however, cross a line that seems farther out of bounds. David Olson was suicidal, in a hospital. His psychiatrist tried repeatedly to recruit him into clinical trials of a new drug. Indeed, drug companies paid his doctor thousands of dollars for each patient the doctor recruited. But David refused to be a test subject. His doctor discharged him from the hospital. He committed suicide two weeks later.

The state medical board found the doctor had "failed to appreciate the risks of taking Patient 46 off Clozaril, failed to respond appropriately to the patient's rapid deterioration and virtually ignored the patient's suicidality." David's sister, Susie Olson, said the doctor "had no time for my brother unless David agreed to get into a drug study. He said, 'You're wasting my time and the hospital's.' It was all about money."

This doctor was not a marginalized "bad apple." He was the president of the Minnesota Psychiatric Society. Many other disciplined doctors also received thousands of dollars from drug companies. An analysis reported by Gardiner Harris and Janet Roberts in the *New York Times* found the drug makers gave a total of $1.7 million to 103 Minnesota doctors who had been formally disciplined by the state medical board, over the period from 1997 to 2005. Presumably the drug makers had also given money to other doctors who had not been formally disciplined.[16]

This poses a particularly tough issue for patients; neither we, nor our doctors, are likely to want to talk about this. If you feel pressured to participate in a clinical trial of a new drug, you can ask who makes it, and later ask the office manager in confidence if the doctor gets money from that company. You can then decide whether you want to continue the relationship with that doctor.

It's rare to be asked to join a clinical trial. More commonly, a doctor might hand you free samples of a drug, with a prescription for more of the same. You can ask if there's a generic equivalent and can emphasize that you'd always prefer generics, wherever possible. You can also privately ask the office manager which drug companies provide free samples to your doctor, and whether those companies have given gifts, speaking honoraria, or nice trips to the doctor. If the doctor later prepares to give you a prescription for those drugs, you can first ask questions about the evidence of the drug's superiority over a cheaper alternative.

You may doubt the doctor's opinion for much more prosaic reasons. Perhaps you've been to a doctor and you're not sure what to do now. Maybe you've received a diagnosis you doubt. Or you've heard you should have surgery but are skeptical. If so, get a second opinion promptly. Dr. Peter Pronovost explains why:

> *"My father died at age 50 of cancer. He had lymphoma. But he was diagnosed with leukemia. When I was a first-year medical student, I took him to one of our experts for a second opinion. The specialist said, 'If you would have come earlier, you would have been eligible for a bone marrow transplant, but the cancer is too advanced now.' The word 'error' was never spoken. But it was crystal clear. I was devastated. I was angry at the clinicians and myself. I kept thinking, 'Medicine has to do better than this.'"*[17]

Dr. Pronovost, now a nationally respected patient safety expert, learned from this awful experience, which fuels his passion. John James similarly channels his energy to save others in health care crises. He says:

> *I lost my 19-year old son several years ago in Texas due to multiple medical errors. He had collapsed while running, self-recovered, but was taken by ambulance to a hospital in his college town. There cardiologists evaluated him for five days and could not find any cause of his collapse. They delegated his follow-up to a physician in training in family medicine, she gave him a clean bill of health, and two weeks later he collapsed and died while running.[18]*

> *As Julia Hallisy, DDS, wrote in her book* The Empowered Patient: *never trust your heart to a single cardiologist; get a second opinion.[19] I would add: make certain it is an independent second opinion rendered without knowledge of the first opinion.*

SUPPLEMENTAL SYSTEMS

In addition to finding an empathic doctor who respects your values and intelligence and has the technical knowledge you need, it's also important to find one who supplements their own knowledge and memory with routine systems. For example, on my way out after a visit with my dentist, his office manager routinely schedules the next visit and has me address a postcard to myself. He keeps the postcard in his desk, amid others that are sorted by the date of the upcoming visit. A few days before the next visit, I get the postcard reminder in the mail: he has remembered me. No computer system is needed.

The cards are often humorous, reminding me of the dentist's gentle sense of humor. So this personalized reminder card system contributes, a little, to my relationship with the dentist. It also yields revenue for him: the reminder cards make it more likely that his patients will show up for their billable visits.

A computer, of course, can do this more elaborately, via the electronic health record – like the one my dog has. I periodically receive postcards from our veterinarian. One featured a photo of a beagle puppy lying down, underneath a golden kitten, and they're looking at each other, nose to nose. Under the title, "Keep your Companion Healthy," are four bullet points: Bring them in for regular exams; Keep their vaccinations current; Ensure a proper diet and exercise; Give them lots of love. On the other side of the postcard is the veterinarian's address and phone number, and a list of the five vaccinations that my dog Jackson should get, with the date that each is due. The message at the bottom says: "Your pet's health is very important to us. Please call for an appointment."

In addition to automatic reminders, the doctor should have a system for routinely providing you with tailored printed or written instructions on your follow-up care – like Jackson's veterinarian does. On the way out, we receive a neatly formatted, five-page summary of the vet's well-dog visit. A paragraph on each of 12 of his body systems describes his condition, with recommendations where needed. Both the dates and reasons for future blood tests and specific immunizations appear at the end. Since the oral exam had detected a tartar build-up on Jackson's teeth, the written recommendations specified the diet, the toothbrush kit (preferably using poultry-flavored toothpaste), and the ideal kind of dog biscuits. The summary appears in the appendix.

A dog's life is easy. For humans, life is harder. Few of us have doctors who provide such information or who now can provide it. Automatic reminders of upcoming visits are more common, even if they often occur through impersonal pre-recorded phone messages. In a few years, many more doctors will have this capability, as the use of electronic medical records spreads throughout physicians' practices. Until then, choose an empathic doctor with the technical knowledge you need.

It's also important to find a doctor who routinely uses safeguards in treatment. It's hard for doctors to remember all the drugs each of their patients takes. Computers, on the other hand, remember everything. Electronic prescribing and order entry systems and pharmacy computer systems contain warnings of dosage errors and drug interactions, and they supplement the doctor's memory, as pharmacists and nurses can do. If a doctor uses neither fellow clinicians nor electronic systems as safeguards, their human - and fallible - memory will sooner or later fail, harming their patients.

> ✚ Have a professional patient advocate help you choose a doctor who uses electronic safeguards and a system of reminders for upcoming visits and diagnostic tests like Pap smears, colonoscopies, etc.

Ideally you can find a doctor who has set up his office with your comfort in mind, as my dentist has done. When I check in for a visit, he walks into the hallway to greet me and ushers me into the exam room with a joke or a smile. When I first met him, he asked my favorite music. So as I settle into the reclining chair for the exam, he selects a CD of my favorite music, which plays throughout the visit. As the chair angles backward, I see above me posters of ocean and tropical scenes and giant hot air balloons on the ceiling, which he has placed there to relax patients. He has designed the space to be consistently relaxing at a time when many people would be anxious.

> ✚ Share this story with your doctor's office manager and ask if there's anything she can do in that way.

YOUR PROFESSIONAL PATIENT ADVOCATE CAN:

- Help you choose an empathic doctor who uses electronic safeguards and a system of reminders of your upcoming needs, via their connections and on-line databases.

- Ascertain the patient satisfaction rates of various doctors in informing your choice among them.

- Find a doctor who'll treat you, rather than treating your lab numbers, and one who is an unusually good listener.

- Ensure the physician you choose has adequate professional backup.

1. AstraZeneca description of Diprivan (propofol), at www1.astrazeneca-us.com/pi/diprivan.pdf and Archibol, R. C., "Michael Jackson's Doctor Is Charged With Manslaughter", New York Times, Feb. 9, 2010, and Coroner's Report, Case Number 2009-04415, available at www.thesmokinggun.com/archive/years/2010/0208101jackson17.html
2. Joshua Perper, "Investigative Report in the Death of Vickie Lynn Marshall (aka) Anna Nicole Smith," BCME# 07-0223, Feb. 8, 2007, pages 12-13. "Dozens of Drugs," Associated Press, Boston Globe, Aug. 11, 2010.
3. Rachel Reid, et al., "Associations Between Physician Characteristics and Quality of Care," Archives of Internal Medicine. 2010;170(16):1442-1449, September 13, 2010.
4. www.SuperDoctors.com
5. Cover pages of the annual "Best Doctor" issue of D Magazine, 2005-2009.
6. Consumer Reports, www.consumerreports.org/health/doctors-hospitals/surgeon-ratings/ratings-of-bypass-surgeons.htm? , Sept. 7, 2010.
7. Katie Smith Milway, "Surviving the incurable cancer," Needham [MA] Times, April 10, 2008, page 15; and Wikipedia.
8. George Reskakis, "To Treat Properly, First Deal with the Fear," NY Times, Nov. 18, 2008.
9. Jerome Groopman, How Doctors Think, New York: Mariner Books, 2007.
10. Stephen Bergman, "The patient is the word," Boston Globe, July 27, 2009, page A13. Reprinted with permission.
11. Bernard Lown, The Lost Art of Healing, NY: Ballantine Books, 1999, pages 17-18.
12. Interview of March 29, 2007.
13. Richard Ferri, "Never Be a Good Patient," Richard's POZ blog, March 25, 2009, at http://blogs.poz.com/richard/archives/2009/03/we_are_not_our_numbe.html Reprinted with permission.
14. Denise Grady, "Foreign Ways and War Scars Test Hospital," NY Times, March 29, 2009, pages A1, A14 and A15.
15. Susan Salladay, "Ethical problems: Pre-op comedy routine," Nursing2008, July 2008, page 60.
16. Gardiner Harris and Janet Roberts, "After Sanctions, Doctors Get Drug Company Pay," NY Times, June 3, 2007, page A1.
17. Claudia Dreifus, "A conversation with Dr. Peter J. Pronnovost," NY Times, March 9, 2010.
18. John James, A Sea of Broken Hearts: Patient rights in a dangerous, profit-driven health care system, Bloomington, IN: Author House, 2007.
19. Julia Hallisy, The Empowered Patient: Hundreds of life-saving facts, action steps and strategies you need to know. Bold Spirit Press, 2008, ISBN-10: 0615177913.

CHAPTER THREE
Choosing Surgery

He was a heavy drinker, and after many years of great stress in his job, and all the vodka, his heart had suffered. Now at age 65 he was running for re-election as the first president of Russia. Boris Yeltsin had had a heart attack and now was experiencing chest pain. He seemed to need coronary bypass surgery, but a Russian surgeon doubted that he would survive the operation.

Accustomed to being a powerful man, Yeltsin was clearly an empowered patient. He asked for a second opinion from the highly esteemed Dr. Michael DeBakey. DeBakey was confident that an excellent Russian surgeon, Dr. Renat Akchurin, could perform the operation, after thyroid and other problems were corrected. In addition to the second opinion, other doctors were consulted, and all agreed Yeltsin would have died if he did not have the bypass.

"I'll do what you say if you can put me back in my office," Yeltsin had told Dr. DeBakey. As a patient, Yeltsin "was not as bossy as he was with some of his Russian doctors," DeBakey said, adding, "He didn't get along with some of the doctors there. But he took a liking to me, listened, and that made things much better…He was deteriorating and going into early heart failure. We gave him 10 ½ years of comfortable life."[1]

Few of us can have access to such a team of doctors, or to far-away doctors at the top of their fields. What does empowerment look like for the rest of us? The first thing is to realize that the decision is more nuanced than it might first seem. There are two decisions: whether to have surgery and if so, where, by whom. This chapter discusses the choice of whether to have surgery at all. The next chapter discusses the decisions of choosing a hospital and surgeon.

> *"What does empowerment look like for the rest of us? The first thing is to realize that the decision is more nuanced than it might first seem."*

INAPPROPRIATE HEART SURGERY

Most doctors, and most surgeons, aren't motivated primarily by money. But the financial incentives consistently and silently encourage more surgery. A particularly blatant example of this affected Father John Corapi when he sought doctors' suggestions for his heart condition. The first doctor recommended surgery, and Father Corapi got a second opinion. This differed greatly from the first, and so he got a third opinion. And a fourth, and even a fifth opinion. He was so surprised by these additional opinions that he went to the FBI.

The FBI performed a three-month investigation. They learned that the first surgeon would often perform an angiogram (an X-ray of the heart arteries, using a dye injected through a flexible catheter tube threaded up an incision in the patient's groin). He did so even for patients with ambiguous symptoms with no history of heart disease. If the angiogram was unreadable, or didn't document a treatable condition, the surgeon would perform an intravascular ultrasound, which was a new procedure at the time. Because he would improperly set the gain on the ultrasound too high, the test would imply that a heart artery was seriously blocked. He would then tell the patient that immediate surgery was needed. Most patients agreed. For those who requested a second opinion, the surgeon would refer the patient to another doctor in his own practice, who would confirm the need to operate. The California Medical Board investigated and found the interpretation of tests had been fraudulently performed in order to scare patients into unneeded surgery, at significant financial gain to the surgeons.[2]

An even more systematic practice of unnecessary heart surgery in California caught Ron Spurgeon in its web. Ron was doing yard work and hurt his shoulder. He eventually saw a cardiologist who told him the condition was life-threatening. Four days later, he underwent triple bypass surgery. Because of a concern that the incision in his breastbone might reopen, restrictions on heavy lifting made Ron, a robust 56-year-old man, give up his job at lumber mills, where he had maintained machinery. Two years after his operation, he learned that the hospital's owner, Tenet Healthcare, had billed Medicare for unnecessary heart procedures. Tenet had paid the U.S. government $54 million to settle the lawsuit. The next year, Ron joined 344 other plaintiffs in suing the hospital, along with eight cardiologists and surgeons, for performing unneeded surgery. After outside experts found that surgeons had performed unnecessary surgery on Ron and many others, the defendants decided to pay $442 million to settle the lawsuit rather than letting it proceed to court.[3]

➕ Do your homework and get a fully independent second opinion before major surgery.

ELECTIVE SURGERY TO PROMOTE THE QUALITY OF LIFE

The most old-fashioned source of advice on choosing surgery is word of mouth, so it's tempting to consider patients' testimonials, especially if you hear them from acquaintances. Some patients spread the word widely. Dave Gibson, for example, had laser-assisted (Lasek) eye surgery. His surgeon then offered him a dollar for every email message touting the operation that Dave sent. Dave, a middle-aged actor, remembers thinking that it was an easy source of money and sent 100 email messages. Another patient mentioned in the same *New York Times* article made an online video, for pay, before he had even finished healing. Six months later, he was still undergoing treatment for the surgery and was less than happy with the results. He did not, however, withdraw the video, preferring to keep the money for his glowing endorsement.[4]

➕ Verify that patient testimonials are unpaid.

A more common condition is being very overweight. Some people have tried dieting without permanent success, as they tend to regain lost weight. Many of them have found bariatric surgery appealing. In this operation, a surgeon closes off most of the stomach with surgical staples or a gastric band, so that even a small amount of food becomes sufficient to make the person feel full.

"Aquameliza" describes her experience with this surgery at age 38:

> *As you can see from my stats – not very impressive – no one would be asking me to be the postergirl for the LAP-BAND®. I did not get enough fills early in the process, but believe that I may actually be approaching my sweet spot soon. I have come to realize a few things and wonder if anyone can relate...*
>
> *I became depressed a few months after surgery when it did not fix everything. Now, I am smart enough to know that it wouldn't, but it still happened. As a result, I found myself drinking alcohol because I could*

and as a way of numbing myself. Alcohol passes just fine through the band and has oodles of calories. So do many other things that I should know better than to eat (ice cream, chocolate, etc.).

So, I faced all of this and stopped the antidepressants (yeah, I think they were messing me up more than helping me) and, although I swore that I would never do this again, walked in to a Weight Watchers week one meeting. Yep – accountability – just like at the start of the band process.

I really never thought I would have to do this again, but the band does not fix everything – it really is just a tool.[5]

Her experience is all too common, as about 40 percent of bariatric surgery patients suffer complications within six months, according to a study by Dr. William Encinosa and others. Many become depressed.[6]

> **"If an operation is often performed more than once for a patient, that means relief is temporary, at best. Moreover, that raises the lifetime risk of a complication."**

A more cosmetic form of elective surgery is also frequently problematic. Krista Schell lives in Thornton, Colo., and works for the state government. She had breast enhancement surgery in 2003 by a California doctor. The same doctor performed a second operation that April to replace a deflated saline implant that had collapsed and made her left breast look "hollow." Her implants were still under warranty. In November, she had a third operation, this time by a Denver surgeon, who removed both implants and extensive scar tissue. The implants had also caused rippling, a lump around one nipple, and pain." If you look at the negatives, you would talk yourself out of getting implants," she said.[7]

Many women have shared Schell's experience. About a third of patients had a second operation within four years of their initial surgery, according to a study by Allergan, a maker of breast implants. "Platinum Suzy" needed a series of operations after receiving her silicone implants, and suffering from contracture of the implants. Two doctors told her she had a reaction to the chemicals in the implants. As good news, she says that the vast majority of women get better once the implants are removed.[8]

Surgery is inherently dangerous, of course. Donda West, the mother of rap singer Kanye West, died after breast implant surgery ("mammoplasty") and liposuction. An internal medicine doctor had warned her against the surgery, in light of her heart condition, which put her at risk of a heart attack. West had not received medical clearance (formal approval by a doctor) before the surgery. A state law now protects California residents like her: the Donda West Law requires medical clearance before elective cosmetic surgery.[9]

✚ **Make sure you get your doctor's formal approval before any elective cosmetic surgery.**

Even very healthy younger women face a risk from surgery. Stephanie Kuleba was an 18-year-old with the world by the tail. An athlete, she had a grade point average over 4.0, long blonde hair, a shy smile, and a formal acceptance to the University of Florida, after which she hoped to work as a doctor. However, she died in the spring of 2008 from a reaction to the anesthesia administered during her breast augmentation surgery.[10]

Ladies, there is a vast conspiracy to make you think you are ugly, so you'll buy beauty products and services. One ad in a women's magazine showed a naked woman with the caption, "You know when you get the perfect pair – and we don't mean shoes." I think differently: like babies, they're all adorable.

✚ **Think long and hard before elective cosmetic surgery.**

Patients and their family members often have to be assertive in stating their wishes to surgeons. Brian Brey, the father of a young boy, was assertive, and yet even this was insufficient. His son's testicle had ascended up out of his scrotum and needed to be returned to its rightful place. Brian discussed exploratory surgery, asking many questions of the surgeon. When the surgeon said the testicle would be removed if it was less than a certain size, Brian stated his preference that it be left alone, and the surgeon nodded. However, the surgeon forgot, or changed her mind, and removed the small testicle, saying that it was "clearly in the best interest of the patient."[11]

➕ Before surgery, they'll ask you to sign a Consent Form to show your formal approval for the operation. Above your signature, write the words: "Surgery is expressly forbidden unless ___," filling in your requirements. Initial that and keep a copy.

Norman Slack, an 83-year-old father of two adult sons, was struggling with his gait – his right leg would get wobbly and begin to shake, and he had had some minor falls. His short-term memory was impaired. While being treated for a heart condition in the hospital, an intern surmised he had normal pressure hydrocephalus (slow fluid buildup in the brain), and wanted to start treatment for it right away, thinking it would improve his gait and memory. After his sons investigated the installation of a shunt (a narrow straw-shaped device) to divert the excess fluid, and he agreed, he received one.

Different doctors had disagreed about whether a shunt was advisable, and one of Norman's sons thought it would be unwise. But a favorable video segment made by the vendor, a satisfied patient Norman had met, the spector of requiring a wheelchair if he didn't have the operation, and the other son persuaded him to undergo the surgery. Unfortunately, it left him incontinent, and his walking has further deteriorated, to the point where he sometimes uses a wheelchair. His short-term memory is no better.[12]

Shunts for this condition often don't help. Half of shunt patients develop an obstruction in the shunt, which requires additional surgery. About 10 percent of shunt patients experience a subdural hematoma (bleeding between the skull and brain). About 50 percent of shunt operations are performed on patients who already have had one installed.[13]

➕ If you have a loved one who is has been diagnosed with hydrocephalus, ask about the specific risks described above, and ask about the alternatives of physical therapy, exercise and wheelchairs.

No matter what kind of surgery you're considering, impartial information sources are vital. Find the website of a respected association of patients with that condition. Perform Advanced Google Searches on the Internet among education (.edu) and nonprofit (.org) sites. See if a decision aid is available. To learn from other patients, you can search blogs for "I had shunt surgery" or the like.

Perhaps the single most telling statistic is the fraction of operations that must be redone. If an operation is often performed more than once for a patient, that means relief is temporary, at best. Moreover, that raises the lifetime risk of a complication. In Norman's situation, for example, a patient would face the risk of a subdural hematoma (bleeding in the brain) each time hydrocephalus surgery is performed. In effect, the more times you roll the dice, the more chances there are to get snake eyes.

SURGICALLY IMPLANTED DEVICES

You should exercise extra caution when a medical device is to be implanted surgically. Calvin Timberlake's case is instructive. A middle-aged forklift operator, Calvin had lower back pain and had a Prodisc implanted in his spine, soon after the Food and Drug Administration (FDA) approved it. A Prodisc is an artificial metal and plastic disk that is designed to take the place of a damaged spinal disk. The Prodisc soon came apart and had to be surgically removed – immediately. Calvin has to take medication now to relieve the intense continuing pain. He didn't realize that his surgeon had invested in the Prodisc. He is suing Synthes, the Prodisc manufacturer, but not his surgeon, whom he doesn't blame.[14]

> ✚ Ask your surgeon's office manager if the surgeon has a financial stake in the medical device that you may receive.

In considering surgery that involves the implantation of a medical device, you'll have conflicting desires. You'll want both the most advanced model, and the most reliable one. It may take time for flaws to reveal themselves, and for a pattern of flaws to be detected, so the most advanced device is not necessarily the best. It's particularly important to research these devices because a recent ruling by the U.S. Supreme Court limits the legal liability of the device manufacturers. The Court ruled that if the FDA had approved the medical device before it was marketed, and if the device meets the FDA's specifications, the manufacturers are immune from liability for personal injury.[15]

A pattern of flaws emerged with heart defibrillators, which are implanted electric devices that shock the heart back into its rhythmic beating, after an episode of quivering without beating ("fibrillating"). Doctors find it easier to thread a defibrillator with narrow electric wires ("leads") through a person's arteries, rather than wider leads. So Medtronic developed a defibrillator with narrow "Fidelis" leads. Stephanie Martinson, then a 35-year-old speech pathologist in Palo Alto, Calif., had received a defibrillator with Fidelis leads. Unfortunately, as the device aged, cracks developed in the wires, which blocked or distorted the electrical flow. This sent faulty signals to the defibrillator itself, which caused it to inappropriately shock the heart. It was providing a jolting shock to Stephanie's heart 26 times an hour. In early 2007, she had the device surgically removed – and replaced with another Fidelis lead, which may well become defective too. The manufacturer suspects that thousands of patients received suspect wires.[16]

Hip replacement patients also have frequently experienced the early breakdown of their implanted medical devices. Stephen Csengeri was one such victim. He had expected the new metal socket in his hip to last for 15 to 20 years. But the metal cup moved around inside the hip socket. The socket was separating from the bone, rather than fusing with it, as X-rays showed, causing excruciating pain only months after the surgery.[17]

Specialized databases known as registries are designed to track such problems with medical devices. Automakers have long based their recalls of defective cars on databases like these. We love our cars, and we care about their parts. The U.S. House of Representatives[18], but not the Senate, voted in November 2009 to develop a national registry of medical devices. With such a registry, we could learn about defects in our own installed parts.

> ✚ Before having a medical device implanted, search the Internet to see if a registry, perhaps one outside the United States, describes consumers' experiences with that device. You may need to hire a professional patient advocate to help you find such a registry and to interpret its reports.

The stories here are not isolated examples. A large expert panel has come to a consensus that certain surgical procedures are performed far too often. The National Priorities Partnership of the National Quality Forum recently identified seven surgical procedures as often unwarranted:

- Back surgery
- Coronary artery bypass graft (CABG)
- Hip replacement

- Hysterectomy
- Knee replacement
- Percutaneous transluminal coronary angioplasty (PTCA) stents
- Prostatectomy[19]

It's a shame that in this day and age, when cars on dealers' lots must clearly display their mileage per gallon on a window sticker, and where refrigerators display their Energy Star ratings, surgical operations are arranged with no clear written statement of their effectiveness, likelihood of repeat operations, complication rates, and patient satisfaction levels, not to mention their price. Until the day when a one-page statement clearly explains that, you'll need to do careful homework in reaching the safest decision.

> ✚ Be especially diligent in learning about the complications (unanticipated outcomes) and the alternatives to these surgical procedures. Get a professional patient advocate to help you in this complex decision.

SAYING NO TO SURGERY

People are likely to feel out of control, and somewhat helpless, when told they'll need surgery. What is it like to say "No," or "Not that way?"

One of the nation's best-known doctors has also faced a personal surgical decision. Dr. Donald Berwick, who long led the Institute for Healthcare Improvement, explains how he considered knee replacement surgery. He asked himself, What do I really want? After thinking, he asked, What do I really, *really* want? Finally, after more thought, he asked himself, What do I really, really, *really* want? His very personal answer is that he wants the sense of peace and purity and complete relaxation that he gets at the culmination of skiing cross-country to a remote silent knoll in mid-winter.

He greatly desires that his own knees will get him to the top of that knoll: those are his functional specifications for the results of any medical treatment of his knees. Berwick has osteoarthritis in his knee, the result of botched surgery when he was in medical school, aggravated later by years of jogging. He chose steroid injections instead of knee replacement surgery and has been able to ski since.[20]

For someone with a professional athlete's soul, the surgery decision can comprise a very different set of considerations than those of a recreational skier. Yena Marcovicci played in the professional tennis circuit many years ago. He kept to a difficult training regimen, running marathons to give him excellent stamina. Late in life, he remained in top condition, competing nationally in tennis against other men in their sixties. He worked as a sports psychologist, and taught the joyous and unforgettable Dance of Tennis class during summers at the Omega Institute in Rhinebeck, N.Y. He died in the prime of his exuberant life at 62 of a heart ailment he knew about but had kept private. He had known his treatment options, and yet chose not to have surgery. Just as the boxer Rocky Marciano decided to retire undefeated in his prime, Yena's decision was consistent with his values and his conception of what his life should be: full, active, joyous, virile, unencumbered by physical limitation. I don't have to agree with his decision to admit, reluctantly, that it was the right decision for him.

You're not likely to have Yeltsin's self-confidence, or Don Berwick's, when considering surgery. Instead, doubt and fear are more likely. I certainly felt that when considering surgery. My primary care physician had referred me to an ENT (ear, nose and throat) surgeon because I was so congested. The surgeon recommended surgery, as they usually do. I checked out of the public library a book about my sinus condition, written by the surgeon who had pioneered the particular operation I was considering. He now performs far fewer of them, having learned that surgical patients usually need repeat operations every few years. In my case, an inexpensive prescription nasal spray makes me much less congested, and has so far avoided the need for surgery. I emailed my primary care physician to discuss that as an alternative, and its dosing and side-effects. He approved of that, after warning of some possible long-term side effects of the drug. Knowing of that possibility, I experimented with taking the drug less frequently, getting his approval to do so, and learning that the less frequent use of the medication still provides satisfactory results. I raise this as an issue at each yearly physical exam, to ensure the plan remains sensible.

So far, this has worked fine, and I breathe comfortably. The medication is far cheaper than the cost and hassle of missing a week from work during the recuperation from the surgery, not to mention the substantial cost that the insurance company would have had to pay for the septoplasty operation.

✚ "Knowledge is the enemy of fear," as the Israelis say. You should quickly try to learn as much as you can about the surgery that is recommended and about your alternatives, and you'll feel much more in control. Begin with Wikipedia to get an overview of your condition, if necessary. But don't stop there. Ask your librarian for help in finding reputable print and electronic sources of information.

I'm more aware than most people of the need to do this, based on the experiences of my large circle of friends and family. A friend's father, as described above, is now incontinent after a "successful" shunt operation to drain fluid from his brain. A close friend had unnecessary cervical surgery after a lesion that was mistakenly thought to be "pre-cancerous" was found. A close friend's father-in-law – himself a doctor – suffered a rare and permanent loss in the body's sense of awareness of where one's hands and feet are ("proprioception") after a surgical error.

Don Berwick and I, like many other health care professionals, consider surgery with a healthy skepticism. Another example is a drug rep, a salesperson who had talked with many doctors in her day. The story of "Shelly," a middle-aged mother of two, appears in an excellent book by Rosemary Gibson and Janardan Prasad Singh, *The Treatment Trap*.[21]

Shelly's doctor diagnosed her as having uterine fibroids (non-cancerous tumors in her uterus), and told her the only option was a laparascopic hysterectomy (camera-guided removal of the uterus via small incisions). Though two other doctors in the practice agreed, Shelly suspected the doctors had a conflict of interest: they would make money only by performing the procedure, giving them a strong financial motive for recommending surgery. Instead, she found a pleasing, less drastic alternative that has left her uterus intact. "It's not enough for patients to know treatment options and their risks and benefits," she says. "You have to understand the business of health care."

These stories and personal experiences, along with the many accounts of medical errors that I have described in the Patient Safety Blog, have made me acutely aware of the gap between what patients seek and what they get. I respect doctors greatly. Some of my best friends are doctors, and I respect my own primary care physician's judgment. But it's only logical that you have to test and question the advice even of a wise advisor who knows you well; you wouldn't take that advisor's suggestion blindly. And you shouldn't blindly accept the suggestion of a surgeon.

> ✚ When your primary care physician refers you to a surgeon for a consultation, do your homework in advance. Identify what you'd like to be able to do afterward, as Berwick did. Find out the alternatives to surgery. Write your key questions, e.g., about how many patients are satisfied with their surgical results, how many can perform the functions you hope to get, how many need subsequent operations, the fraction who have complications, and how many similar procedures that surgeon has performed. Bring someone to the surgical consultation with you to record the answers, as your advocate can hear more calmly and fully than you will.

FINDING AN ALTERNATIVE FORM OF SURGERY

A systematic search process should be helpful, like the one Terri Nelson performed. Her doctor had diagnosed fibroid tumors and scheduled a follow-up visit with her surgeon for two weeks later. During that time, she and her husband industriously researched her condition and the most common treatments. She started with the authoritative Mayo Clinic and Pub Med websites. Then she reached out to the online community of fibroid patients.[22] Panning through the huge river of online information "to find the nuggets of valid information in the sea of online hypochondria," she found a blog for the layperson, "Inquisitive Geek with Fibroid Tumors."[23] By the time she saw the surgeon, she knew some of the side-effects of the traditional treatment of hysterectomy and a surgical alternative ("myomectomy") that leaves the uterus intact. She was able to discuss that, and choose it, with the surgeon.

For many conditions, there are clear, unbiased and very authoritative materials, both printed and on compact discs, which are available through the non-profit Foundation for Informed Medical Decision Making.[24]

> ✚ After a systematic search like the Nelsons', talk to individual patients who have confronted the choice you face.

The decisions against surgery are examples of the conscious and idiosyncratic choices of knowledgeable, empowered people. A decision to have surgery, even when not recommended by a doctor, can reflect a similarly knowledgeable, thoughtful choice.

Bonnie Denis was only 3 years old when a rare virus, transverse myelitis, attacked her central nervous system. It left her temporarily paralyzed below the waist. But she bounced back quickly, and by age 5, "I was doing handstands on my walker." But as she grew, the muscles in her feet atrophied, and the bones grew crooked. Now, when she walks, it feels "like there are a bunch of knives stabbing me," she says.

Even so, she has lived a very active life, dabbling in acrobatics. She keeps an active and quirky sense of humor. At 30, she made a difficult and rare choice, after many operations and years in a wheelchair. The decision is as personal and unique as her custom-painted, raspberry-pink crutches. She decided to find a doctor to amputate her excruciating right foot.

The decision follows a series of operations. While she was in high school, surgeons invented a series of procedures to reshape her feet. They broke bones and reset them. They implanted metal pins and took them out again. They augmented her own bones with bones from cadavers. Once horrified, she came to think it's cool: "I'm part zombie," she says.

Bonnie knows the trade-offs; she knows surgery, and wheelchairs, and what it feels like to walk. She is making her own choice – maybe not the one you or I or her doctors would make for themselves – but it's a well-considered decision, and it's hers.[25]

> ✚ Make your own decisions on surgery after careful consideration and consultations.

YOUR PROFESSIONAL PATIENT ADVOCATE CAN:

- Help you identify your ultimate health goal and consider the trade-offs of alternatives for reaching it.

- Research the success rates for the type of surgery you're considering and identify and describe your alternatives to surgery.

- Accompany you to the surgical consultation and clearly hear what the surgeon isn't saying.

1. Lawrence Altman, "The Doctor's World:In Moscow in 1996, a Doctor's Visit Changed History," NY Times, May 1, 2007.
2. Gerald Rogan, Frank Sebat and Ian Grady, Disaster Analysis Redding Medical Center Congressional Report, June 1, 2008.
3. ---, "Treatment traps to avoid:
Insured? You're money in the bank to the health-care system," Consumer Reports Health.org, November 2007.
4. Abby Ellin, "Coming Soon to YouTube:My FaceLift," NY Times, June 26, 2007, pages E1 and E3.
5. Blog post atwww.lapbandtalk.com Jan. 29, 2009.
6. Encinosa WE, Bernard DM, Chen CC, Steiner CA. "Health care utilization and outcomes after bariatric surgery," Medical Care. 2006 Aug;44(8):706-12.
7. Natasha Singer, "Do my breast implants have a warranty?", NY Times, Jan. 17, 2008, pages E1 and E3.
8. Email communications, March 15, 2008 and March 23, 2008.
9. Karen Bonsignore, K.J. Matthews and Lola Ogunnaike, "Coroner awaits toxicology test results in death of Donda West," CNN.com, Nov. 13, 2007, and Wikipedia article on Kanye West.
10. Tanya Rivero and Jonann Brady, "Florida Teen Dies After Complications During Breast Surgery:Doctors Believe a Reaction to Anesthesia May Have Caused Death," Palm Beach Post, March 25, 2008.
11. Brian Brey, personal email message of April 4, 2009.
12. Email communication from Kim Slack, May 11, 2010.
13. Codman & Shurleff, Inc., Life NPH website: www. lifenph.com/surgery.asp Nov. 26, 2010.Also, see Hydrocephalus Association website: www.hydroassoc.org/
14. Reed Abelson, ""Financial Ties Cited as Issue in Spine Study," NY Times, Jan. 30, 2008, pages A1 and A14.
15. Linda Greenhouse, "Justices Shield Medical Devices from Lawsuits," NY Times, Feb. 21, 2008.
16. Barry Meier, Barnaby Feder, and Lawrence Altman, "Heart Devices Encountering a Blind Spot," NY Times, Oct. 16, 2007.
17. Barry Meier, "The Evidence Gap:A Call for a Warning System on Artificial Joints," NY Times, July 29, 2008.
18. See www.PatientSafetyBlog.com/2009/11/suffering-they-save-may-be-their-own.html re H.R. 3962.
19. National Priorities and Goals:Aligning our Efforts to Transform America's Health care, Washington, DC:National Quality Forum, 2008.
20. Robert Pear, "Obama Chooses Health Policy Scholar as the Director for Medicare and Medicaid," NY Times, March 27, 2010, and ""Patient-Centeredness and Patient Safety: How Are They Interconnected?", a presentation by Donald Berwick, Boston, September 17, 2009.
21. Rosemary Gibson and Janardan Prasad Singh, The Treatment Trap:How the overuse of medical care is wrecking your health and what you can do to prevent it, Chicago: Ivan R. Dee, 2010.
22. John Schwartz, "Surfing for a Second Opinion," NY Times, Sept. 30, 2008.
23. http://blog.geekwithfibroids.com
24. Foundation for Informed Medical Decision-Making website: www.informedmedicaldecisions.org/patient_decision_aids.html
25. S.I. Rosenbaum, "Her argument for amputation," Boston Globe, June 16, 2008.

CHAPTER FOUR
Choosing Your Hospital and Surgeon

In the 1950s he had recorded dozens of Top 40 songs, including the number one hits, "Wish You Were Here," "I'm Walking Behind You," "Oh! My Pa-Pa," and "I Need You Now." He was also known for marriages to Debbie Reynolds, Elizabeth Taylor and three other women.

Eddie Fisher died on September 22, 2010, after complications from hip surgery at a hospital in Berkeley, Calif.[1]

"Complications" is a euphemism for additional problems that arise following a medical procedure, treatment or illness and are related to that.[2] It's always plural, which hints at the deliberate vagueness or knottiness of the idea. Some of every hospital's patients experience complications, but the rates vary greatly. Rarely, hospitals' rates of complications are made public.

Around the time of Eddie Fisher's demise, one of the glamorous and beautiful women he didn't marry – Zsa Zsa Gabor – experienced declining health. At age 93, she had fallen, breaking her hip in July 2010. She had hip replacement surgery in Los Angeles, and then had to return to the hospital the next month to remove the blood clots that later developed.[3]

If you don't know a hospital's rate of complications for a procedure you're considering, the best you can do might be to find a surgeon – and a hospital – that perform many of those procedures. There's a learning curve for operations, as for everything else in life: practice makes less imperfect.

The reason you should choose a high-volume surgeon and hospital, of course, is because they have learned from their experience at perform-

> *"The reason you should choose a high-volume surgeon and hospital, of course, is because they have learned from their experience at performing that specific procedure."*

ing that specific procedure. Each time they see a patient for follow-up, they learn something about what worked well or poorly. They get muscle memory. They learn from their mistakes at the hospital's morbidity and mortality conferences. They have hobnobbed more with colleagues who perform those procedures and have learned from their stories.

Unfortunately, there are no guarantees. Eddie Fisher had treatment at a community hospital; Zsa Zsa Gabor had been treated at a teaching hospital that probably had much more experience at hip surgery. Both had poor outcomes. The best you can do is to maximize your chances.

> Look at the publicly available information to compare at least three hospitals in your area at www.HospitalCompare.hhs.gov. This excellent source of data clearly reports everything from patients' opinions to indicators of quality and mortality rates for many kinds of medical and surgical care.

"Hundreds of thousands of Americans travel abroad for healthcare each year. Now, universal health insurance may make that largely unnecessary."

If there is a specialty hospital that performs the procedure you need, try to get treatment there. That's also the recommendation of Dr. Peter Cram, the lead author of a study of more than 1 million Medicare patients who received hip or knee replacement surgery. His team found that surgical patients at specialty hospitals experience 40 percent fewer blood clot, bleeding, infection, and fatal complications than patients at community hospitals.[4]

Look for a surgeon who has performed many of those procedures. Denise Grady of the *New York Times* tells the story of a relative who learned she had rectal cancer and would need surgery, radiation and chemotherapy. She first consulted a kind local surgeon, who doubted he could save the sphincter muscles that make it possible to control one's bowel movements. She would likely need to permanently wear a colostomy bag to divert her wastes. Instead, she found a surgeon who specialized in rectal cancer. Today, she's in good health, with no colostomy bag.[5]

Denise's relative was lucky in that the first surgeon took the time to fully inform her about the risks of surgery. When she later consented to surgery with another surgeon, hers was fully informed consent. "Informed consent" is required, but is only rarely genuinely obtained. In practice, the patient is asked, seemingly as a formality, to sign a lengthy, informed consent form using language they may not understand, often without much real explanation of the risks and benefits of surgery. Until a law is passed requiring disclosure of the effectiveness and complication rates, you should ask for them, while realizing that your surgeon may not know the answers.

While in the hospital, of course, patients experience much more than just the surgical procedure itself. Along with the larger number of nonsurgical patients, they receive medication before and after the surgery, information on follow-up care, lab tests, X-rays, MRIs and other imaging tests, diagnoses, special diets, and much more. Each of those is subject to error – indeed, sometimes to fatal error. Many of those errors can be prevented by computerized physician order entry (CPOE) systems. For example, one study found that CPOE systems reduced medication errors by two-thirds.[6] CPOE systems act as umbrellas that prevent a wide variety of errors. They can prevent overdoses and underdoses, inappropriate drugs, mistimed drugs, and mix-ups of patients, among many others. The more sophisticated CPOE systems prevent diagnostic errors through their "clinical decision support." So it's important to find a hospital whose physicians routinely use a CPOE system. Some hospitals already have them in widespread use; others are in earlier stages of their use, and some hospitals are even slower. A recent federal law gives hospitals financial incentives to reach a level of "meaningful use" of CPOE systems. However, very few (14 percent, according to a recent study) will have reached that by the deadline in 2011.[7] Full implementation throughout the U.S. is likely to take many years. Most community hospitals lack CPOE systems, though they are more common among teaching hospitals.

✚ Seek a hospital with an active CPOE system in wide use by calling the hospital's risk manager beforehand.

Here's an example of how one woman who's not a celebrity, but should be, sought and found excellent hospital care. My mother has always put her family members' concerns ahead of her own, which sometimes comes at her own expense. In September 2009, our whole family assembled for my teenage daughter's bat mitzvah, a Jewish coming-of-age ceremony. Not wanting to hog my daughter's spotlight on her special day, my mother waited until the morning after the event to tell me that she was feeling pain radiating down her neck. Fearing it might be a stroke, I had to decide promptly where to take her. Within a half hour drive of our home in suburban Boston are several teaching hospitals. I called two of the nearest ones and asked their waiting times as of that moment. I knew the main sites of the teaching hospitals in Boston proper, about a half hour away, would likely be busier than the smaller ones nearby. Upon learning that there would be no wait at the nearest teaching hospital, Beth Israel Deaconess Medical Center's Needham Campus, I obtained their ER's fax number and drove to the hospital. While on the road, I called my mother's primary care physician's office in Atlanta and had them fax her problem list and medication list to the ER as background information.

My mother tells the rest of the story:

> *Ken had encouraged me to go to the ER even though I didn't want to, since later that afternoon I was going to Connecticut to see some old friends. It was a pleasant surprise to be taken immediately; I'd expected the usual two to three-hour wait in an emergency room. I had a series of tests that included an EKG, blood work and X-rays.*
>
> *People were friendly and efficient, and quick, so by the time I was lying in the special room they put me in, the next thing I knew a neurologist was speaking with me from the screen, and I had no idea where he was from. It was very strange to be able to converse back and forth. He could ask me questions and I could ask him questions, two-way communication, which was a new experience – it was really amazing. I expected somebody to just come in and introduce himself and say goodbye.*
>
> *I was really impressed with the speed with which they got the results from the tests. By the time I was finished with all the tests, the neurologist on the TV screen [in Boston] had the results available to him. That was amazing! By the end, they were able to say for sure that it wasn't a TIA [a mini-stroke, or transient ischemic attack]. I was merrily on my way to see my friends in Connecticut, and was even able to catch the same train I'd made a reservation for! I was so impressed that everything went so quickly and so smoothly.*

> *Since everything had been computerized at my Atlanta hospital – Wesley Woods, the geriatric division of Emory Hospital – they could fax it to the hospital in Needham immediately. If they had still used a paper system, my information might have been misfiled, or might not have been available right away to be faxed.*

In the recent past, many Americans who had meager or no insurance and faced very costly surgery became "medical tourists" who sought and underwent less expensive operations abroad. Patient Safety Blog reports stories of satisfied patients who received care in China, Costa Rica, India, Israel, Mexico, Switzerland and Thailand. Hundreds of thousands of Americans travel abroad for health care each year. Now, universal health insurance may make that largely unnecessary.[8]

> ✚ If you urgently need very expensive surgery and don't yet have health insurance, carefully consider finding a surgeon and hospital in another country. You'll need a professional patient advocate to help you with this complex decision.

YOUR PROFESSIONAL PATIENT ADVOCATE CAN:

- Help you find the best surgeon.

- Help you find the safest hospitals by referring to various databases.

- Consider all the pros and cons of getting medical care abroad.

---

1. Robert J. Lopez, "Eddie Fisher dies at 82; popular singer known for high-profile marriages," Los Angeles Times, Sept. 24, 2010. Eddie Albert's songs: Wikipedia
2. Complications definition: www.MedTerms.com
3. CBS News, "Zsa Zsa Gabor in 'Extremely Serious Condition'," August 15, 2010, at www.cbsnews.com/stories/2010/08/15/entertainment/main6775508.shtml
4. Peter Cram, "Specialized Hospitals Seem to Have Lower Complication Rates," University of Iowa Health Care Today March 2010, at www.uihealthcare.com/kxic/2010/03/orthopedic_surgery.html
5. Grady, Denise, "Should Patients Be Told of Better Care Elsewhere?," NY Times, Jan. 6, 2009.
6. Bates, DW, Teich J, Lee J, Seger D, Kuperman GJ, Boyle D, et al., "The impact of computerized physician order entry on medication error prevention," J Am Med Informatics Assoc 1999; 6: 313-321.
7. Jason Hess et al., "CPOE Digest 2010: Traffic Jams on the Road to Meaningful Use," KLAS Research, 2010.
8. Paul Keckley, "Medical Tourism: Consumers in Search of Value," Deloitte Center for Health Solutions, 2008.

CHAPTER FIVE
In the Hospital

Professional Patient Advocates should have protocols they'll follow, step by step through a patient's hospitalization. The stories and suggestions in this chapter will supplement, rather than substitute for, detailed protocols.

I still remember the helpless fear I felt on a bus in 1978 as we twisted our way along the narrow hilly road leading to Jerusalem, steered by a sleepy bus driver. Each time he nodded off, his head then snapped right up again. Thank God, we arrived safely.

But God didn't prevent an accident from exhaustion when my son was born, 12 years later. Going into premature labor eight weeks early, my wife was admitted to a Harvard teaching hospital, where doctors delayed her childbirth for a week. They gave her beta dimethasone, a drug to speed the maturation of the lungs of our unborn baby. Two days later came one of the happiest days of my life, when we learned that a lab test revealed the drug had worked: my son's lungs would be fine, and he wouldn't need a ventilator.

Residents had affixed a band and device around my wife's belly to measure and graph the fetal heartbeat and the contractions of her uterus. Noticing the graph showed regular peaks, I asked a young resident what that meant. She reassured me that it was fine, and I didn't pursue it.

Then when hearing in the evening that my wife was experiencing abdominal pain, the sleep-deprived residents confidently attributed them to gas pains. Finally, the next morning a pelvic exam revealed her cervix was nearly fully dilated, ready for delivery. Exhaustion had ruined their judgment, so my wife had had to suffer labor pains for 12 hours without any pain medication.

> **"We both respected the knowledge of our young doctors, and were horrified at the effects of their exhaustion and group-think."**

The doctors at the Harvard teaching hospital had missed the fact that my wife was in labor. They'd ignored their device, ignored my question about the rhythmic spikes in uterine contractions, and misdiagnosed my wife's pain. Luckily, my son was born very healthy.

And yet, we're grateful to the doctors for effectively using the drug that magically reached my son's lungs. The care they provided was both miraculously better than our expectations in one way, and stupid in another. We both respected the knowledge of our young doctors, and were horrified at the effects of their exhaustion and group-think.

> ✚ Respect your doctors' knowledge and always stay vigilant – before you enter the hospital, in having a diagnostic work-up, before and during surgery and other procedures, and on going home.

This chapter discusses what to do at each of these times, in turn.

BEFORE ENTERING THE HOSPITAL

Ed Bradley, the long-time CBS News journalist best known for *60 Minutes*, lived for years with leukemia, after a quintuple bypass.[1] Hopefully he had the support of friends and family when he needed them. Patients with very taxing diseases can use lots of help with meals, shopping, getting to doctor's appointments, etc. An excellent free resource for organizing and contacting supporters during a health crisis appears on the Internet at www.LotsaHelpingHands.com. As this is also very helpful for people with chronic conditions, an example of its use appears in Chapter 9.

> ✚ Patient advocates should organize helpers by using that website in advance of a hospital stay, so the help can begin promptly when the patient returns home.

ON ENTERING THE HOSPITAL

Famous people may get better care in the hospital, but even they are not immune to infections. CBS newsman Ed Bradley died in a hospital from an infection. It was never made clear whether the infection had been acquired in the hospital, or outside it. The star quarterback of the New England Patriots, Tom Brady suffered a staph infection following his knee surgery[2]. Twenty-year-old Brazilian beauty queen Mariana Bridi da Costa died of blood poisoning (septicemia) after a urinary tract infection, as mentioned in a previous chapter.[3] More recently, U.S. Congressman John Murtha had a surgical infection during his gallbladder surgery and died soon afterward.[4] Thousands of lesser-known Americans die each year from hospital-acquired infections.

Nurses, doctors and other staff in hospitals are becoming much more aware of hospital infections. Yet some still don't wash their hands often enough or take other precautions. The mindset is still not good enough. Consider hospital scrubs – those distinctive, simple, usually blue, shirts and pants that doctors and nurses wear while in the operating room. Wearing scrubs became a badge of the profession, like wearing a white coat or carrying a stethoscope. Since then, it has become a fashion statement to wear scrubs outside, e.g., while shopping in the supermarket. Now it connotes high tech, medical science, good health, saving lives, and looking like Dr. Meredith Grey or Dr. Preston Burke.

Scrubs are characteristically made of cotton. Now there are also scrubs made of blends of polyester and cotton to maintain "a wrinkle-free professional looking appearance with little fuss."

A few years ago, I once hung out on Longwood Avenue in Boston, near several Harvard teaching hospitals, with two Australian friends, as they laughed uncontrollably every time they'd see a doctor or nurse on the street in their scrubs. Then I got it: An urban street is far from sterile. If scrubs mean, "We're taking special care to be sterile," then why are clinicians wearing them on the street? Just because it's easy, to look cool, and announce their status (and announce they're not keeping them sterile)? Will they wear the same scrubs in the OR? They've become their opposite. While your nurse friends may look great in scrubs like mine do, seeing them should warn you that their workplace and the staff themselves are much germier than they look.

While they get to look really cool in their scrubs, they dress us patients in gowns. I like to look silly – once in a great while, at Halloween. But even then, I don't cross-dress. I don't do dresses. Or nightgowns, negligees or chemises. And the thought of those ridiculous gowns with a drawstring that opens in the back, and the little tchotchke designs, makes my skin crawl.

So at a recent emergency room visit, I brought my blue terrycloth bathrobe and wore that. This seemed to give conniptions to the ER nurse, however, and I didn't want to appear as a uncooperative patient, so I gritted my teeth and put on the johnny. I'm in good company, as Don Berwick concluded his essay on the meaning of patient-centered care by saying, "what chills my bones is indignity....It's the image of myself in a hospital gown, homogenized, anonymous, powerless, no longer myself."[5]

> ✚ You can reduce your embarrassment while wearing a johnny by imagining that the doctor or nurse examining you is wearing only a flimsy gown with a drawstring that has come open in the back.

A Boston radio station aired a story on a Harvard teaching hospital, where a nurse observed staff on the cardiac unit to see who was washing their hands and when.[6] What makes the nurse sure that they won't know they're being watched? Oh, she has taken off her name tag – but still wears the standard blue nurse's uniform and white coat. For 10 minutes, she notes who washes their hands. Meanwhile, the cardiac unit nurses hurry around the unit, probably aware of the one nurse, not from their unit, who isn't hustling around. Surprise! Everyone dutifully uses the hand sanitizer while she watches them. Does this spot-checking really raise compliance with hand-washing rules? Or does it just provide a reassuringly high rate of hand-washing?

A more reliable approach uses unobtrusive measures to give a more honest, untainted view. At Beth Israel Deaconness Medical Center in Boston, for example, staff instead measure the volume of hand sanitizer used. They track the total volume of use over time to determine whether overall use is increasing or decreasing.

> ✚ Bring a bottle of hand sanitizer and leave it on the table in your hospital room as a gentle reminder for clinicians to wash their hands.

You should also bring some other important materials, as the next story suggests. An 85-year-old man with severe psoriasis was admitted to the hospital because he had been experiencing confusion, forgetfulness and weakness over the last three weeks. His medication list included oral methotrexate, 25 milligrams every Saturday at breakfast and lunch. Before dispensing any methotrexate from the hospital pharmacy, the pharmacist recognized that a 50-milligram weekly dose seemed high and asked the nurse to confirm it. The patient verified that that dose was correct. A second pharmacist also questioned the order and called the patient's family, asking them to read aloud from the prescription container. The dose of the drug the man had been taking at home was 2.5 milligrams. The pharmacists had intercepted a would-be 10-fold overdose error.[7]

✚ Bring all your medicines to the hospital with you. If you have an updated list of the drugs and doses, bring that too.

DIGNITY AND PRIVACY

We're all infatuated with celebrities. I had a huge crush on Farrah Fawcett. We used to watch her TV show, *Charlie's Angels*, though we kept the volume off because the dialogue was so insipid. She beautified my brother's college dorm room wall, which boasted the iconic poster of her smiling, seated, in a red bathing suit, with her golden hair cascading everywhere.

Many years later, Fawcett became very ill with cancer and received treatment at UCLA Medical Center. She suspected that hospital staff were leaking her records to the press because so many stories were being published about her condition. To test that, when she learned about a specific recent diagnosis, she delayed telling her family. When a story about the diagnosis appeared in the press, that proved that a hospital employee had been snooping and had leaked the story.

A low-level employee had viewed Fawcett's records on 104 days in a 10-month period in 2006-07. That employee later pled guilty to federal felony charges of selling the information about the star and many others to the *National Enquirer*.

But other snooping employees were not punished so severely. California health regulators eventually learned that 67 other employees of UCLA Medical Center had snooped into the care that Fawcett, Britney Spears, Tom Cruise, Mariah Carey and other celebrities received.[8]

✚ The federal government aims to protect patients' privacy in the HIPAA law (Health Insurance Portability and Accountability Act). On the HIPAA form your provider gives you, write in restrictions on who can access your medical records.

DIAGNOSIS IN THE HOSPITAL

Tyler Kahle was a 19-year-old youth who lived in Omaha, Neb. In the fall of 2002 he had chest pain, which brought him to the hospital twice, and to his doctor's office once, in an eight-day span. Doctors diagnosed it as an upper respiratory problem, and sent him home. They disregarded his mother's comment that the family had a history of aortic dissection (a tear in the lining of the artery that takes blood from the heart). They never ordered a scan that would detect that.[9] This dangerous condition is treatable, and can be fatal; in fact, it took the life of actor John Ritter.[10] Tyler died four days after his second hospital visit.

✚ If you doubt a doctor's diagnosis, ask what else it could be. If you know an inheritable condition may be involved, ask if that can be ruled out as a diagnosis, and on what basis.

John Ritter was best known as a star of the TV sitcoms *Three's Company* and *8 Simple Rules for Dating my Teenage Daughter*. The circumstances around his aortic tear were very different, as he and his family, unlike Taylor's parents, were unaware of the risk he faced. He had been told to see a doctor for his heart condition several years earlier but hadn't done so. Then, in February 2008, an aortic tear happened too quickly for doctors to intervene in time. His widow had brought a lawsuit alleging that doctors missed the diagnosis, and that an X-ray could have detected the condition, allowing for treatment. The jury, however, disagreed, finding that the doctors could not have prevented Ritter's death. Perhaps Ritter himself could have prevented the condition, but wasn't mindful of the need, early on, to see a doctor.

A technique to repair such heart arteries had been developed long ago by surgeon Michael DeBakey, back in 1954. At first, he used a Dacron tube he'd made on his wife's sewing machine. Fifty-four years later, at age 98 he became the oldest survivor of the procedure he invented:

Never had a symptom. The pain came like a bullet out of the blue. I was alone when it started. My wife and my daughter had gone out. The pain is often described as the worst pain you can have. The pain was so severe that I would have welcomed anything to relieve it – including death. I wasn't going to fight it. I look upon death as a part of living, just as some trees lose all their leaves in the winter and have them replaced in the spring. But at the same time, part of me was thinking, what caused this pain?

Part of me was doing a diagnosis on myself – which, as it turned out, was correct. Aortic dissection. I'd written more articles about the condition than anybody in the world, and I resigned myself to having a heart stoppage. The pain didn't teach me anything about the heart. It simply emphasized what I had already learned.

I was a little surprised to find myself recovering after the surgery, then gratified to have been given a second life.

During my recovery, I played possum. I pretended to be sleeping and listened to what the doctors standing over my bed were saying about my condition. Then I'd argue with them about the therapy. I'd make them prove I needed it. I guess it's hard to be my doctor.[11]

Of course, if you're not an expert, this strategy of playing possum and then arguing with doctors is not advisable.

> Yet you certainly can ask for a satisfying explanation of what your doctors are recommending, and why. You can say, "Can you please explain that? What will I need to do afterward to get back to being 100 percent healthy?" Better yet, get an advocate to be with you through this difficult time. That's important because it's very hard to think clearly when you're fearful or anxious. An advocate will be calmer and more experienced in these situations.

HOSPITAL TREATMENT

The less you speak "medicalese," the more important it is to get a professional advocate. One Spanish-speaking woman sought surgery in Massachusetts for trigger finger, a condition where the finger catches in a bent position and straightens with a snap. The surgeon signed his name on the correct side of her body, to prevent wrong-side surgery. However, the woman received carpal tunnel surgery on her wrist instead of surgery on her finger. For this patient, the Spanish/English language barrier contributed to a serious error. That hospital has since set a policy of making interpreters available during surgery on non-native English speakers.[12]

> If a family member doesn't speak English, insist on having an interpreter or advocate nearby before surgery so your family member will fully understand and agree with the procedure.

Of course, it might be that your family member can't communicate for other reasons. If that's the case, you'll need to be extra vigilant. You may notice signs that even nurses don't, as Myra did, in this story about her mother:

> *My mom went through a rather "interesting" few days. She was in the hospital overnight on Thursday for symptoms of a TIA, discharged on Friday, and doing very well Saturday morning.*
>
> *They were all set to go out after lunch, and then she just got weak, couldn't walk, and had to be carried to bed. The nurse checked her out and vitals were fine. She slept all afternoon. But by 4:00 Guy and the aide got more concerned when they couldn't rouse her. By the time I got over there around 5 p.m., she had a severe headache, slurred speech, and a weak left side.*
>
> *We called an ambulance and when she got to the ER, I suggested they start an IV of fluids. They disagreed. Instead they did a CAT scan and an EKG. Both normal. They gave her a Tylenol for her headache, which did nothing. By 10 p.m. she was screaming in pain, confused and agitated, and they gave her a shot of morphine. By the time the needle left her arm, she was sound asleep and peaceful. She was admitted to a room after midnight and had a pretty good sleep. I once again suggested an IV of fluids, but the nurse did not think that Mom was dehydrated.*

On Sunday they did an MRA (as opposed to an MRI) and an EEG and both were negative for stroke and seizure. They did labs and ruled out infection. They decided to cut back on her blood pressure meds because her blood pressure was also low.

I went home on Sunday around noon while Guy stayed for the afternoon and we had a private aide for overnight. On Monday morning, the aide reported that Mom had a terrible night, did not sleep, and the headache was back. When I got there around 10:30, her speech was slurred and she was listing over to the left. A hospitalist came and decided to order an IV of fluids. I waited with her all afternoon, and she fell sound asleep – so deeply that once again she could not be roused: not by yelling at her, rubbing her arm, or pounding on her chest. However, the IV never came and the nurses and PT just thought she was having a "sleepy" day. Ridiculous.

By 5:00 pm I insisted that a doctor see her again and that the IV be started immediately. They started the drip at 5:30 and at 5:40 her eyes fluttered open and she started to revive. They ran the drip all night long – I slept over again – and by this morning she was bright, perky, and not (too) confused. Speech and strength on both sides were normal. Headache gone. She walked with her walker and held court with the various staff members!

I took her home at 2:30 and when I left at 4:00 she was busy making dinner plans with friends for this evening and trying to decide on what kind of little celebration she should have for her upcoming birthday. I asked her if she wanted to nap and she was not a bit sleepy. I was really stunned that dehydration (plus, low blood pressure probably) could cause these kind of severe complications.[13]

✚ If exercising that degree of vigilance is difficult, as it is for most people, look for a professional patient advocate. See Chapter 12 to learn how they help, and how to find a good one.

The more esoteric the treatment, the more you'll need a professional advocate. For example, some new radiation treatments are quite complex and lack built-in safeguards, making them risky, as this story shows:

Scott Jerome-Parks was raised in a conservative family in Gulfport, Miss., later moving to Toronto, and then New York City. There, he met his Canadian-born wife, Carmen, a dancer, singer and aspiring actress. He took a job as a computer and systems analyst at the southern tip of Manhattan.

Haunted by the deaths he saw up-close on September 11, 2001, he volunteered to work with the Red Cross near "the Pile." He developed what he initially thought was a nagging sinus infection, diagnosed two months later as tongue cancer. His doctor believes there was a link between his tongue cancer and the toxic dust from the collapsed towers, though the cause of his cancer was never proven.

Scott approached his illness as any careful consumer would, evaluating the treatment options before choosing a hospital. He chose a hospital that provided Intensity Modulated Radiation Therapy (IMRT), which it advertised as more precisely targeted, and so having fewer serious side effects, than conventional radiation therapy.

"The next day, she died from complications in the surgery. Actually, she had not had cancer. The hospital laboratory had mixed up her pathology report with another woman's."

The first four radiation treatments had been provided as prescribed. The medical physicist revised the treatment plan for the fifth session to better protect Scott's teeth from radiation damage, at the suggestion of Scott's doctor. Such a revision of the treatment plan is a time-consuming task. As the medical physicist tried to save the computer program containing the revised treatment, late in the morning of March 14, 2005, the system crashed after appearing to save the changes first. An hour later, Scott's doctor approved the new plan. Half an hour later, the computer crashed again. Six minutes later, staff administered the first of several radioactive beams. They administered another round the next day.

Two friends – a layman and a nurse – noticed something wrong because of Scott's intense pain, and swelling throughout his head and neck, and asked the hospital to check on Scott. They sent a psychiatrist. Scott received another round the next day. Several hours later, the medical physicist ran a test to see whether the radiation had been provided appropriately. Then she tested again, and tested a third time. A frightful mistake had been made: Scott's entire neck had been exposed, causing a large overdose of radiation. The damaged cells were not reparable. Scott died in early 2007 at age 43.

The New York City hospital treating him for tongue cancer had failed to detect a computer error that directed a linear accelerator to blast his brain stem and neck with errant beams of radiation. Not once but on three consecutive days. In an exceptionally thorough data analysis, the *New York Times* found that the complexity of this new technology has created new avenues for error – through software flaws, faulty programming, poor safety procedures, or inadequate staffing or training.[14]

➕ For patients undergoing radiation, your advocate should insist on a test of the equipment by a medical physicist before the radiation is applied. The test is customary but is sometimes skipped in the interest of time, as it was here.

BEFORE SURGERY

Make sure every nurse and doctor knows your first and last name. They should start by greeting you by name. If they don't, shake their hand and introduce yourself. If you don't, you risk getting the wrong operation. That's very rare, but it does occur. Here's an example of a switch that occurred at a hospital in Somerville, Mass., in November 2005:

Two patients with the same first name were waiting in the gynecological clinic, in nearby exam rooms. One needed a colposcopy – an examination and biopsy of the vagina and cervix. The other woman needed a routine, less-invasive checkup. While hanging the charts outside the exam room doors, a medical assistant accidentally switched the women's charts.

One woman mistakenly received a colposcopy. The chief of surgery later stated that neither she nor her interpreter had objected.[15] Perhaps they didn't object because they didn't know exactly what the procedure would entail. In general, it's helpful to learn ahead of time what steps your procedure will involve. That way, you may know enough to ask the doctor a question before it's too late.

For this purpose, and in the general spirit of patient education, some hospitals equip patients with a specific description of the care they will receive. For example, cardiac patients at Massachusetts General Hospital in Boston get a care map – a "Patient Pathway" schedule – that shows patients the procedures and milestones in their cardiac care.

Surgeons often depend on X-rays in deciding whether to perform surgery. In the case of "Sofia" this decision was more complex than it appeared at first:

Sofia is an active 79-year-old girlfriend and grandmother of four, an ex-skier from the days when young women didn't ski. Back then, she had broken her leg on the ski slopes. Now, with no reason, she suddenly had developed excruciating pain while walking.

She called her doctor, who had her come in to see a colleague who was covering for him while he was out. The covering doctor admitted her immediately to the local community hospital in suburban Connecticut. There, based on her X-rays, a surgeon prepared to operate the next day on her hip fracture. The surgeon planned to install three screws in her right hip to stabilize it.

Sofia's family prepared for a difficult operation and a lengthy and painful recuperation. Then, suddenly, the next day, they received a phone call: there was no hip fracture. Two of the three X-rays had found nothing, and the third had found a line suggesting a possible fracture. This is not uncommon, as X-ray interpretation is very subjective. Radiologists will disagree on about a fifth of all X-ray films.[16] The surgeon had ordered an MRI, which clearly found no fracture. Sofia scooted out of there as fast as she could.[17]

✚ **Get a fully independent second opinion on X-ray readings before surgery if there is any doubt of their interpretation.**

Sometimes lab test results can be very clear, and yet very wrong in another way. In the spring of 2007, doctors at a hospital on New York's Long Island told a 30-year-old woman they had detected cancer in her left breast. Because of her family history of breast cancer, she chose to act swiftly and decided on a double mastectomy. The next day, she died from complications in the surgery. Actually, she had not had cancer. The hospital laboratory had mixed up her pathology report with another woman's, according to an investigation by the New York State Department of Health.[18]

✚ Read the test results yourself before surgery and verify that the report shows your name and date of birth.

Indeed, you should verify more than just your name and date of birth. You should read your medical chart itself to prevent wrong-site surgery, as this story proves. In late 2007, the Rhode Island Department of Health reprimanded and fined one of the state's hospitals for its third wrong-site surgery of the year. In this case, a CT scan had shown bleeding on the left side of the brain of an 82-year-old man. Staff brought him to the neurosurgical intensive care unit for brain surgery. A resident (a physician in training) began drilling into the right side of the man's brain. When the intern realized the mistake, he closed the incision and performed the operation on the left side.[19]

✚ Require the attending physician to accompany a resident anytime you have surgery. A teaching hospital may allow residents to perform certain surgical procedures. You should write onto your patient consent form that your entire surgical procedure must be performed by an attending physician rather than a resident alone.

Immediately before surgery, within the hour before surgery, nurses often administer a prophylactic antibiotic, i.e., to prevent a hospital-acquired infection. Make sure this is done, and if it has not been done, verify that that was a deliberate decision that you understand and agree with.

VIGILANCE DURING THE HOSPITAL STAY

One of the most preventable causes of death in the hospital is "failure to rescue." That refers to cases when caregivers do not notice or respond in time when a patient is dying of preventable complications in a hospital. Between 2004-2006, 188,000 inpatients died in these circumstances.[20]

A few hours before cardiac arrests and respiratory arrests, certain warning signs usually occur. If someone detects and acts on these warning signs via a "Rapid Response Team" or "Rapid Response Method," doctors and nurses can usually prevent a cardiac or respiratory arrest. If these signs are not noticed and heeded, cardiac arrests (when the heart stops) and respiratory arrests (when breathing stops) usually bring resuscitation attempts (e.g., in a Code Blue), but these attempts usually fail.

"A trigger [for a Rapid Response Team] is not about excitement and drama; it's about intervening before there's drama," says Jeanne Quinn of Beth Israel Deaconess Medical Center in Boston. A senior nurse with 15 years of experience, Jeanne had participated in a rapid response for Carol Emerson, who was in the hospital for the repair of broken bones in her arm. Emerson's blood pressure had plunged to 56, so her less-experienced nurse had activated a trigger for a rapid response. A sudden decrease, or increase, in blood pressure, or a sudden sustained increase or decrease in pulse or heartbeat, or confusion, are the body's warning signs that a cardiac or respiratory arrest may be imminent. Responding within minutes, Jeanne helped the nurse gradually restore Carol's blood pressure into the 100s. The team ordered an electrocardiogram and a blood transfusion, and they kept Carol in the hospital an extra night – alive.[21]

It's impossible to know whether this rapid response prevented a cardiac arrest. In general, with the benefit of hindsight, about half of hospitals' rapid responses are warranted, according to one study.[22] That rate of valid alarms (true positives) is so high that clinicians are generally very supportive of policies and criteria about calling for rapid responses.

Otherwise, all too often, no one heeds the critical warning signs. "As an example," says Dr. Samantha Collier, the chief medical officer of HealthGrades, "somebody comes in for elective knee surgery like a knee replacement and turns up with vague symptoms, like shortness of breath, and the next thing you know, somebody dies. It's obvious that if you go in for knee surgery, you shouldn't die."[23]

Of course, even highly educated and caring doctors and nurses aren't perfect, so it's critical that family members also stay vigilant, and be willing to insist on a rapid response when needed. In Massachusetts, South Carolina and some other states, state law explicitly authorizes family members to call for a rapid response. In any event, the body that accredits hospitals – the Joint Commission on Accreditation of Healthcare Organizations, or JCAHO – also explicitly required hospitals to heed a family member's request for a rapid response, as in its National Patient Safety Goal #16.01.01.

I've led the Rapid Response Work Group of the Consumer Health Quality Council, within the parent Health Care for All organization. In that role, and my role as president of the Council, we have been gathering statistics on family members' calls for rapid responses. We have identified only a smattering of such calls during 2009; exceedingly few family members called for rapid responses. Few know they can do so. With better education and publicity about this, they'll be able to safeguard their loved ones in the hospital.

✚ It's vital that family members should stay vigilant and call for a rapid response if you're in doubt.

On the other side, there are some times when a hospital patient's condition is deteriorating, such that family members prefer that doctors and nurses not intervene. As Kathleen Kalt explained:

> *More patients need to know that they do not have to comply with every doctor's request. My daughter had leukemia at age 10 and clear-cell sarcoma at 17. She was treated by outstanding doctors, but we all knew she would not survive the second cancer. When she had to be admitted to a major teaching hospital for surgery, it seemed she was on all the Grand Rounds; everyone wanted to see this rare case and hear her medical history. We didn't think she needed to relive constantly the worst moments of her life. She needed dignity and control. We gave our own orders: "No one will touch her except her primary doctors. She won't answer any more questions. Read her chart for yourself." After seven years dealing with the medical establishment, we knew that the best patients were their own advocates.*[24]

✚ To preserve your child's dignity, you can give your own orders to guide the learning of interns and residents in the teaching hospital. It's best if you put them in writing and sign it, telling both the attending physician and nurse manager, and asking them to include your note in the medical record.

These difficult situations are discussed further in Chapter 8, Coping with Grave Illness.

GOING HOME: UPON DISCHARGE

When you're ready to be sent home, have a friend or family member help you. Particularly if it's soon after you've had conscious sedation, this is important, as your judgment may be impaired in some subtle ways.

Before my own procedure under conscious sedation under Versed and Fentanyl, nurses appropriately told not to make any important decisions later that day. I felt quite in control afterward, however – which was quite a deceptive feeling. I had no memory, for example, of having written a thank-you note to the doctor, or of asking someone to pass my note to the doctor afterward.

When George W. Bush was president, Vice President Richard Cheney was once temporarily in command of the United States, during President Bush's colonoscopy. The president, we were told, had the minor outpatient procedure under conscious sedation, and handed over command to the vice president for a few hours. The procedure removed five polyps from the president's colon before they could become dangerous. The president resumed his duties a few hours later.[25] That poor judgment placed us all at risk. Fentanyl is deceptive in leaving people falsely feeling that they are in complete control.

> ✚ Have a companion help you for the rest of the day, after you've had conscious sedation for a hospital procedure. Don't make important decisions during the rest of the day.

If you don't have a friend or family member who can help you, or if you anticipate that life will be very difficult for you after you're discharged from the hospital, you should ask the hospital discharge planner if the hospital has social workers or counselors who might help. For example, such staff can help match you with an insurance company and help you identify government resources that you qualify for, like food stamps, housing assistance, Social Security disability coverage, and many other social services. They might help you find a primary care physician if you don't have one.

Francine Fitz, for example, benefited from such a counselor. A telemarketer, widowed and approaching her 60s, she lives in central Massachusetts. She couldn't afford her employer's health insurance plan, as she was earning about $10 an hour. A counselor at the University of Massachusetts Medical Center helped her find both insurance and a primary care physician so she could see her own doctor, and stop going to the emergency room, for routine medical care.[26]

Of course, there are no guarantees that the recommendations made in this chapter will save your life. But all of them are free, safe and sensible.

CHECKLIST FOR PATIENT ADVOCATES

Respect your doctor's knowledge and always stay vigilant – before you enter the hospital, in having a diagnostic work-up, before and during surgery and other procedures, and on going home. You may need a professional advocate for many of these tasks.

BEFORE HOSPITALIZATION

- Bring a bottle of hand sanitizer and leave it on the table in your hospital room as a gentle reminder for clinicians to wash their hands.
- Bring all your medicines to the hospital with you. If you have an updated list of the drugs and doses, bring that too.

IN THE HOSPITAL

- On the HIPAA form your provider gives you, write in restrictions on who can access your medical records.
- If you doubt a doctor's diagnosis, ask what else it could be. If you know an inheritable condition may be involved, ask if that can be ruled out as a diagnosis, and on what basis.
- Ask for a satisfying explanation of what your doctors are recommending, and why. You can say, "Can you please explain that? What will I need to do afterward to get back to being 100 percent healthy?" Better yet, get an advocate to be with you through this difficult time.
- If a family member doesn't speak English, insist on having an interpreter or

advocate nearby before surgery so your family member will fully understand and agree with the procedure.

- Get a fully independent second opinion on X-ray readings before surgery if there is any doubt of their interpretation.
- Read the test results yourself before surgery and verify that the report shows your name and date of birth.
- Require the attending physician to accompany a resident anytime you have surgery. Write onto your patient consent form that your entire surgical procedure must be performed by an attending physician rather than a resident alone.
- For patients undergoing radiation, the advocate should insist on a test of the equipment by a medical physicist before the radiation is applied.
- Call for a rapid response if your loved one's condition deteriorates.
- You can give your own orders to guide the learning of interns and residents in a teaching hospital. Write them and sign them, telling both the attending physician and nurse manager, and asking them to include your note in the medical record.

AT DISCHARGE FROM THE HOSPITAL

- Have a companion help you for the rest of the day after you've had conscious sedation for a hospital procedure. Don't make important decisions during the rest of the day.

1. ---, "Admirers to Pay Final Respects to Bradley," from BET.com News Staff & Wire Services, Updated Nov. 21, 2006.
2. Shira Springer, "Infection Slows Brady's Rehab," Boston Globe, Nov. 11, 2008, page C1 and C8.
3. Shari Roan, "Beauty queen's amputation is rare complication of septicemia," Los Angeles Times, Jan. 23, 2009.
4. Carol Leonnig and Paul Kane, "John Murtha's condition is 'stable' and 'improving' as he battles infection in ICU, sources say," Washington Post, Feb. 3, 2010, at http://voices.washingtonpost.com/44/2010/02/john-murtha-in-stable-conditio.html?wprss=44
5. Don Berwick, "What 'Patient-Centered' Should Mean: Confessions of an Extremist," Health Affairs, May 9, 209, pages 555-564.
6. Sasha Pfeiffer, "Rapping Nurses? Boston Hospitals Launch Creative Hand-Washing Campaigns," WBUR, aired June 2, 2009, at www.wbur.org/2009/06/02/hand-hygiene
7. Michael Cohen, "Don't cheat the order sheet," Nursing2008, June 2008, page 23.
8. Charles Ornstein, "More tied to UCLA snooping," Los Angeles Times, May 12, 2008, and Charles Ornstein, "Kaiser hospital fined $250,000 for privacy breach in octuplet case," Los Angeles Times, May 15, 2009.
9. Michael O'Connor, "Hospital offers rare mea culpa after death," Omaha World-Herald, Aug. 29, 2007.
10. ---, "Ritter's doctors cleared in wrongful death case," ContactMusic.com, Feb. 28, 2008 and Mar. 15, 2008.
11. Cal Fussman, "What I've Learned: Michael DeBakey [interview]," Esquire, March 2008, page 182. Reprinted with permission.
12. Stancel Riley, Jr. et al, "Massachusetts Department of Public Health Patient Safety Update: Wrong-Site Surgery," 2009, at www.mass.gov/Eeohhs2/docs/dph/patient_safety/wrong_site_surgery.pdf
13. Email message from patient advocate Myra Fournier, March 10, 2010.
14. Walt Bogdanich, "A Lifesaving Tool Turned Deadly," NY Times, Jan. 24, 2010.
15. Liz Kowalczyk, "Surgical mistakes persist in Bay State," Boston Globe, Oct. 26, 2007, page B1 and B8.
16. Jerome Groopman, How Doctors Think, Boston, Houghton Mifflin, 2008, page 181.
17. In-person interview with respondent, March 2007.
18. Cara Buckley, "Long Island Hospital Is Investigated after Patients' Deaths," NY Times, Feb. 11, 2008.
19. Liz Kowalczyk, "R.I. raps hospital for errors in surgery," Boston Globe, Nov. 27, 2007, page B2.
20. HealthGrades.com-in-the-news, 2008.
21. Liz Kowalczyk, "Hospitals Try to Break a Deadly 'Code,'" Boston Globe, Nov. 27, 2005.
22. Institute for Healthcare Improvement, IDS White Paper: Reducing Hospital Mortality Rates, Part 2, at www.ids-healthcare.com/Common/Paper/Paper_53/Reducing%20Hospital%20Mortality%20Rates%20%5BPart%202%5D.htm
23. HealthGrades.com, ibid.
24. Kathleen Kalt, Letter to the Editor, NY Times Magazine, May 6, 2007.
25. Jim Rutenberg, "Bush has 5 polyps removed in colon cancer test," NY Times, July 22, 2007.
26. Kay Lazar, "Costly E.R. still draws many now insured," Boston Globe, Oct. 6, 2008, pages A1 and A7.

CHAPTER SIX

In the Mental Health World

"Normal" is someone you don't know very well, as Elizabeth Lesser says in her memoir.[1] We're all quirky, all somewhere along a very broad and wildly colored mental and behavioral health spectrum. Indeed, the "bible" of the psychiatric profession – the DSM IV[2] – now lists more than 400 different neuroses, psychoses and other psychological conditions. Most of us fall into at least one of those categories, which include everything from academic problems (Code V62.3) to voyeurism (Code 302.82).

These forms of dysfunction are often not objectively ascertainable. Detecting and identifying them can be tricky, and their treatments usually rely on professional judgment as much as on hard evidence. In this subjective and personal realm, friends, family members and neighbors have an especially strong role in identifying the need for treatment and for starting and continuing treatment – even more so than for more purely physical conditions. Only a small fraction of people with mental and behavioral health problems get treatment for them, and many will only begin treatment if a family member or close friend leads them in. The stories in this chapter describe how friends, family members and professional advocates have helped get people into treatment, and out of inappropriate treatment.

GETTING INTO TREATMENT

In the behavioral health world, providers say that we heal in groups. We're umbilical beings; we get nourishment from others in many ways, long after leaving the womb. Many people who use drugs and alcohol do so, in effect, to treat themselves for depression or loneliness. Advocates can help get people into a wide range of types of treatment. Some of them are described here, from the most familiar to least familiar.

> *"We're umbilical beings; we get nourishment from others in many ways, long after leaving the womb."*

COUNSELING

Professional advocates serve a matchmaking function, getting a client into appropriate treatment. Sometimes treatment starts only long after the trauma. It took Madison, N.C., resident Peter Griffin nearly 30 years to receive the medals he earned in Vietnam and just as long to acknowledge something he brought back with him from the war – post-traumatic stress disorder (PTSD):

"I was 17 when I joined and only 18 when I shipped out to Vietnam," he said. "Combat is difficult enough for hardened veterans, but so many of us in that war were still just teenagers." Peter served with the 101st Airborne Division and the 82nd Airborne Division. He earned the Vietnam Service Medal with two bronze battle stars, the Silver Star Medal, the Army Commendation Medal, the Presidential Unit Citation with oak leaf cluster and the Valorous Unit Citation.

Later, as a civilian policeman, he was injured in a fall from a roof while chasing a suspect. At a Veterans Affairs hospital for a checkup, he discussed with doctors the other symptoms he was experiencing. He sought out a Department Service Officer (DSO), James Ward, while trying to get the Silver Star he earned during a battle in Vietnam. When Ward asked him to describe the incident in which he earned the medal, Peter became agitated and began having flashbacks. The DSO recognized his symptoms and encouraged the veteran to let him file a claim. "I told him I didn't want him to do it because I didn't want to be labeled with another disability," Peter said. "Fortunately for me, he didn't listen." A call from a VA hospital and a series of tests from doctors and psychologists confirmed the DSO's suspicions and set Peter on a course of treatment to conquer the demons with which he had long lived.

PTSD is an extreme anxiety disorder resulting from psychological trauma. Peter wrote his story in a book in the hope that "it will be a help to others out there suffering through the same hell I was going through."[3]

THE MEDICAL HOME

That gentle persistence shown by Peter's DSO is matched by Sori Santana, in this story by Dr. Heidi Behforouz:

> *Sori Santana is one of my PACT [Prevention and Access to Care and Treatment] community health workers. Sori told the story of Maria. A young woman with significant mental illness, and a cocaine user, Maria was referred to PACT with her immune system ravaged by uncontrolled HIV. For four years, Sori rode life's ups and downs with Maria, always encouraging, never forcing. Yet she was never able to help Maria consistently take her medications. Then one day, something clicked. Maria began taking her pills. She's now getting stronger and has voluntarily taken on the role of accompanying her boyfriend, showing up in his room with a cup of coffee in one hand and his psych pills in another, telling him that if he doesn't get up and take his meds, she is going to "pull a Sori on him."*
>
> *With the power of such accompaniment, we have documented significant clinical improvement in the majority of our patients and reduced preventable hospitalizations by 40 percent. We have been creating – to borrow a phrase – patient-centered medical homes. Much of the care is being delivered by paraprofessionals who have not been extensively schooled in the biomedical model and don't practice office-based care. Their schooling and expertise is in the art and science of "accompaniment" – you walk with the patient, not behind or in front of her, lending solidarity, a shoulder, a sounding board, a word of counsel or caution. Empowering, not enabling. Together facing and managing challenges that neither you nor they can fix – poverty, racism, illiteracy, social isolation – so that you can help them swallow their pills every day, get to their appointments on time, and renew their Medicaid applications.*[4]

✚ Professional advocates like James Ward and Sori Santana can help find treatment options and accompany people into them.

BRIEF HOSPITALIZATION

Cheryl [not her real name] is a middle-aged mother with an adult son and daughter. She graduated from an Ivy League college and ran a small business for many years. Then in midlife she ran into several crises simultaneously. She had spent much more than she could afford; she was undergoing a nasty divorce; and she faced an impossible deadline at work on a make-or-break project for the small company that employed her. The strain was too much, and she told her mother that she felt suicidal. Knowing of my blog and my patient advocacy work, Cheryl's sister contacted me, and I went to help.

Her boyfriend, son and I chose to bring Cheryl to an academic medical center, where she was given a psychiatric evaluation. We chose an appropriate outpatient psychiatric hospital, which provided individual and group therapy and different medications over 10 days. I prepared a set of recommendations for her family to simplify and manage her finances, and to negotiate a more reasonable role at work, and helped them to start implementing the recommendations. Realizing now that her problems couldn't be solved by herself alone, she has been in psychotherapy for the last few months. She returned to her job, mostly enjoying it, and her boyfriend, while living less large. The multiyear divorce proceedings continue to drag on. But for the most part, the crises are behind her.

> *"Advocates will sometimes need to help forestall inappropriate treatment."*

As an advocate, I helped choose and interact with two providers, provided moral support to Cheryl and her family, and made and carried out recommendations to ease underlying areas of stress and to equip her to regain a more stable life.

E-THERAPY

For some people, it's difficult to find a counselor or therapist, perhaps because they live in a remote location. John Khoury describes an innovative alternative at www.liquic.com:

> *Vera [not her real name] was a middle-aged mother in Holland with an alcohol problem. Things got to a point where she needed to see someone. Here in Holland, you first see a general practitioner, and then they send you to a specialist. She'd seen a couple of psychiatrists, but didn't have good experiences with them, and never really got to the question of why she was drinking. Instead, they'd said she just had to stop, in order to have therapy.*

That wasn't going to work. It wasn't the right match; it wasn't a good therapist for her. She found a website of a community forum of people with alcohol problems. In that kind of forum, things can open up a bit. She reached out to an Internet therapist who was specializing in the treatment of alcohol abuse. That clicked very quickly with her; it was a very different experience.

She appreciated the online contact with him. He gave her tips and homework. He didn't insist on abstinence right away. She appreciated that. He would teach her to postpone her drinking. For example, he'd say, Take the dog out for a walk, and then see how you feel 20 minutes later. She hasn't completely stopped drinking, but it's not a problem for her anymore.

Vera preferred that to face-to-face therapy because of lack of time constraints. In face-to-face therapy, you get off on a tangent and then time runs out, and you never get to what you really had in your head to talk about, that you sort of lost track of in the moment. With e-therapy and emails, if a thought is in her head, she writes it down and sends it off to a therapist.

She said "it saved my life," that it has been the thing that made a real difference in her life. Things are smoother with her family, and she has started painting. A positive effect in your life affects the people around you: her husband has stopped drinking so much. There's no going back. It's like in mental health in general: once you feel good, with your head straight on your shoulders, you know how that feels. Then you can repeat that same feeling of mental health.

Since then, Vera wrote a book under a pseudonym in community with these other people. People get friends for life, like in Vietnam Veterans groups. They meet occasionally face to face with each other, and with the therapist. That's a big step.[5]

✚ e-Therapy may be an option when face-to-face counseling isn't available or appropriate.

GETTING AWAY FROM INAPPROPRIATE TREATMENT

Advocates also need to intervene if there is too much treatment. To a man with a hammer, everything looks like a nail. Psychiatrists and psychotherapists may see mental illness when it's not there. Advocates will sometimes need to help forestall inappropriate treatment.

The world of behavioral health providers seems divided into the haves and the have-nots. The have-nots include drug and alcohol counselors, and many, if not most, psychotherapists. These providers work in nonprofits or small practices and typically regard money as dirty. They're rarely wealthy. They often have a personal history of behavioral health issues in their families, which inspires a deep sense of commitment. Psychiatrists, with medical degrees, occupy the other end of the income continuum. Many work for large hospitals and drug manufacturers. While many of them are committed members of helping professions, their corporate cultures often socialize them to promote their services and drugs, sometimes at the expense of patients. The active marketing of the big pharmaceutical firms, and the medicalization of ordinary conditions, have created an environment where mental illness may well be greatly overdiagnosed and overtreated. Medical doctors have legal authority to write prescriptions and commit patients to mental hospitals, and many other powers, and they drive the bus.

Nowadays, teenagers are not merely "rebellious" pains in the neck; rather, they have "Oppositional Defiant Disorder" (DSM Code 313.81), i.e., a medical diagnosis for which they can be profitably medicated for years. Young women with diva personalities are not drama queens; rather they may have "Histrionic Personality Disorder" (Code 301.50). Or perhaps Adjustment Disorder (309.9), Antisocial Personality Disorder (301.7), Communication Disorder (307.9), Disruptive Behavior Disorder (312.9), Expressive Language Disorder (315.31), Impulse-Control Disorder Not Otherwise Specified (312.30), or if not, certainly Disorder of Infancy, Childhood or Adolescence Not Otherwise Specified (313.9).

> ✚ Upon learning of a family member's psychiatric diagnosis, take a walk through the DSM IV, and see how many diagnoses would fit you. Then take the diagnoses with a good healthy dose of skepticism, repeating the dose as needed.

The apparent overuse of the new "atypical antipsychotic" drugs offers a case in point. The overuse of psychiatric drugs may be especially severe where there is the least openness, e.g., in jails. A study of the use of atypical antipsychotic drugs in jails in 16 states found that many youths in American juvenile facilities are getting strong antipsychotic drugs for bipolar and schizophrenic conditions, even when they have not been diagnosed with the conditions that warrant their use. "Fifty years ago, we were tying kids up with leather straps, but now that offends people, so instead we drug them," says Robert Jacobs, a former Florida psychologist and lawyer. "We cover it up with some justification that there is some medical reason, which there is not."

In Texas, for example, one-fourth of all the incarcerated youths in Texas in 2008 had at least one prescription for an atypical antipsychotic drug, though 71 percent of them did not have a diagnosis of bipolar disorder or schizophrenia. The state of Texas had formally developed a protocol (the Texas Medication Algorithm Project, or TMAP) to identify the preferred medications for the state's Medicaid and mental health clients. Pharmaceutical companies paid physicians to make presentations touting the benefits of atypical antipsychotic drugs, so the TMAP would encourage their use. The large CATIE study in the U.S, and another study in England, however, had found that the new atypical antipsychotic drugs were no better than the older drugs, though they cost 10 times as much. Dallas newspapers publicized the payments made to influence doctors who were writing the TMAP. A whistleblower, Allen Jones, brought a lawsuit in Texas, later joined by the Attorney General of Texas, against the drugmakers. The lawsuit is ongoing as this book goes to press. Indeed, in recent years, four major drug companies – Bristol-Myers Squibb, Eli Lilly, Pfizer, and AstraZeneca – have settled lawsuits brought by the U.S. government, which accused them of illegal practices related to the marketing and promotion of antipsychotic drugs. Drugmakers had used a similar process in Pennsylvania and many other states to promote state committees' formal approval of the wide use of atypical antipsychotic drugs.[6]

✚ **Carefully consider the side effects and alternatives to psychoactive drugs.**

Hospitalization for mental illness can also be inappropriate at times. In Joseph Heller's novel, *Catch 22*, the protagonist, bombardier Captain Yossarian, learns that:

There was only one catch and that was Catch-22, which specified

> *that a concern for one's safety in the face of dangers that were real and immediate was the process of a rational mind. Orr was crazy and could be grounded. All he had to do was ask; and as soon as he did, he would no longer be crazy and would have to fly more missions. Orr would be crazy to fly more missions and sane if he didn't, but if he was sane he had to fly them. If he flew them he was crazy and didn't have to; but if he didn't want to he was sane and had to.*[7]

The mental health world ensnares patients in a similar logic. This story happened to someone I've known for a long time, whom I trust completely. Demographic details are fictitious, but the story is real.

Amanda is a 15-year-old drama queen in New Orleans. She enjoys creative writing and sassing adults. She competes on swimming, soccer and basketball teams, and participates in drama and musical groups at school. These activities give her many friends, whom she keeps up with on Facebook. A tomboy, she has abandoned her wardrobe of camouflage clothing in favor of a slightly Goth look, since it seems to provoke her parents more reliably. She is a vegetarian because she abhors the idea of killing animals.

Faced with a series of tests at school that she considered demeaning, she sought a creative way to refuse to take the tests. She answered the open-ended questions with stories about people dying. Her teachers thought this represented a cry for help and convinced her father to promptly bring her to a mental health crisis center for a psychological evaluation to consider whether that behavior revealed that she might have a personality disorder, e.g., depression or a tendency to harm herself.

At the crisis treatment center, the mental health intake worker performed a pro forma assessment, and indicated that Amanda should be admitted for observation to a psychiatric hospital. The intake worker didn't ask her father the context of Amanda's actions. Amanda was upset at the prospect of being sent to a psychiatric hospital and upset that the intake worker hadn't been listening well. She ran away, despite the torrential rain, getting lost. Realizing she needed help in getting home, she stopped at a gas station and asked them to call the police. The police came and called an ambulance that brought Amanda to the nearest hospital's emergency room.

Her parents hurried to the ER, finding that Amanda was drenched and angry but was otherwise okay. Mildred, another mental health worker from the crisis center, saw Amanda in the ER and tried to have Amanda admitted to a psych hospital for observation. Mildred considered Amanda a "flight risk." To meet the legal requirements for this, a psychiatrist's signature was needed. The signatures had been rubber-stamped onto a set of blank forms so the assistant herself could fill one out to authorize the hospital admission.

The parents objected since the law requires a consulting psychiatrist to order the admission. The father had obtained a blank, signed form and showed it to the ER medical staff, proving that no psychiatrist had been involved. Embarrassed by the obvious short-circuiting of the law, Mildred negotiated with Amanda's parents about the form and extent of follow-up care. The ER physician had been busy with other patients for the first four hours that Amanda was in the ER. Once the ER physician became available, he performed a one-minute assessment that medically cleared Amanda, enabling her parents and their neighbors to take her home. Amanda's parents agreed to phone in daily for three days with the crisis treatment center and to arrange for a therapist to meet with Amanda. They did so. Amanda's weekend, involving two major milestones in a 15-year-old's social life, was wrecked, and she was emotionally distraught, but after a couple of weeks, she said, she had become herself again.

In *Catch-22*, every pilot has to get in the plane and fly, sane or not. In the crisis treatment center world, every client is considered to be a patient, and every patient must be admitted as an inpatient. If the school thought the student was at risk and gets the student to the treatment center, they must have had grounds to think that way, and it would be dangerously irresponsible for the treatment center to allow the student to go home that night. Moreover, the treatment center, of course, makes much more money if they admit the student overnight. If the patient is completely healthy, the psychiatrist's judgment, and observation over 24 hours, will reveal that. And if the patient was completely healthy, she wouldn't be there. So everyone is admitted as an inpatient.

If the staff didn't admit the patient overnight, the school teachers would not feel she was safe. If they didn't feel that referring students like Amanda to that center kept the student safe, they would refer students in the future to a different treatment center. That would lose business for the treatment center. So the incentive is clearly for the crisis center to admit patients as inpatients.

Every assessment produces a decision to observe the patient overnight. Intake staff know that patients are distraught and angry, so patients can't answer responsibly. Nor can the parents. If patients make their explanations calmly, they show a lack of affect, which could be a sign of a personality disorder. If there is a chance they could have a personality disorder, it's best to admit them as an inpatient. If they're angry, on the other hand, they may have an anger management problem, but only observation would allow an accurate diagnosis. If they're quiet and sullen, that could show their anger is turned inward, which is interpreted as a sign of depression, which of course, requires further evaluation. In the center.

Because everyone is admitted anyway, there's really no point in having a real psychiatric consultation when the patient first gets there. It would be a waste of the psychiatrist's time. So the rubber-stamped signature of a psychiatrist is sufficient. And any trained staff member, even a layman, can fill out the admission authorization form above the psychiatrist's signature, because the signature means it was acceptable to the psychiatrist.

At every link in the treatment chain there was a Catch-22. When Amanda left the treatment center, she had asked the police to help her get home. But because she had been at the treatment center, the police had to bring her to the hospital. Being at the treatment center meant to them that there was a chance she could harm herself, so to protect her they had to call an ambulance. Like Captain Yossarian, sane or not, Amanda was getting into that vehicle. Once in the ambulance, she couldn't ask to be taken home. The ambulance only went to the hospital. It would be dangerously irresponsible of them to bring her home, sane or not, healthy or not. And their revenue depended on them bringing her to the hospital; the hospital gives them much or most of their business. Once she showed up at the ER, doctors and nurses there had to assess her. That is their responsibility by law, even if a completely healthy and sane person is brought there. Even if the crisis center had erred and said so, or even if the police had erred and said so, even if the ambulance drivers had erred and said so, the ER staff had a legal responsibility to assess the patient. They could discharge her, but only after medically clearing her, i.e., after their doctor's approval.

This system produced one ruined weekend for Amanda, a lot of agitation for her parents, and bills exceeding $2,000 for crisis treatment, transport by ambulance, and ER treatment. Amanda is as healthy as most other adolescent American drama queens. Her parents induced the crisis treatment center to cover the ER copayment and ridiculously large ambulance fee through a series of certified letters.

The system is designed for erring on the side of caution. And for revenue: Let no one, and no small change, fall through the cracks. The down side is that someone who is falsely suspected of having a mental health issue, and so enters the maw of the mental health care beast, can only be discharged out the other end; there's no other exit from the belly of the beast midway through it.

In the mental health world, providers assume that the clients are mentally impaired. Laws accordingly empower providers to make certain decisions even over the objections of patients. Amanda offers a case in point. Because of this disempowerment of patients, it's likely that errors in treatment may be very common in mental health treatment. Patients may not know an error has occurred or may not be believed when they contend that they've suffered a medical mental health error.

> It's especially important for mental health patients to have an advocate.

YOUR PROFESSIONAL PATIENT ADVOCATE CAN:

- Find treatment options for you and accompany you there.
- See if a medical home might have appropriate behavioral health services.
- Research the pros and cons of different types of treatment for you.
- Help you with re-entry back home.

1. Elizabeth Lesser, Broken Open: How difficult times can help us grow, NY: Villard, 2004.
2. Allen Frances et al., Diagnostic and Statistical Manual of Mental Disorders: Fourth Edition, Washington, DC: American Psychiatric Association, 2000.
3. Peter Griffin, When You Hear The Bugle Call: Battling PTSD and the Unraveling of the American Conscience, Trafford Publishing, 2007; and Steve Lawson, Reidsville Review, Jan. 17, 2007.
4. Heidi Behforouz, "Health Reform Lessons, via Haiti and Peru," Boston Globe, Dec. 21, 2009, page A11.
5. Interview with John Khoury, Feb. 25, 2010.
6. John Kelly, "Psych Meds in Jails," Youth Today, Oct. 1, 2010, at http://youthtoday.org/view_article.cfm?article_id=434; Marian Wang, "In Some States, Incarcerated Kids Get Drugged to Alter Behavior, Despite Risks," ProPublica Blog, Oct. 4, 2010, at www.propublica.org/blog/item/in-some-states-incarcerated-kids-get-drugged-to-alter-behavior-despite-risk ; Emily Ramshaw, "Conflict of interest fears halt children's mental health project," Dallas Morning News, Aug. 18, 2008.
7. Joseph Heller, Catch-22, NY: Simon and Schuster, 1996.

CHAPTER SEVEN
After the Error

You'll feel in shock, and angry. Puzzled. Maybe with a sense of dread. You'll have lost your innocence, and it might seem that nothing will be the same, that this is the first day of a life you didn't ask for and don't want. You'll need to act fast, and that will be nearly impossible. You may feel mad at yourself, at your own inability to prevent this from happening. You'll learn bit by bit over time, and will think differently about the error the month after it occurs, the following month, and in the longer run. Accordingly, this chapter first discusses what to do before the injury, in the moment, before discussing what to do in the medium and longer run, in turn.

BEFORE THE INJURY

You might intercept an error from reaching the patient, preventing injury. For example, a doctor in a hospital might order the wrong dose of a drug, committing an error. But if the pharmacist, nurse, patient advocate or patient realizes the mistake, they can intervene before any adverse consequences occur. Tammy Alvarez of St. Joseph's Hospital in Orange, Calif., describes a similar case in a California hospital in which a patient who was an engineer had handed his nurse a list of his medications for the nurse to copy during the formal routine process of medication reconciliation. She miscopied it, omitting a heart medication. He didn't say anything directly to her but expressed some vague concerns to a doctor. The doctor contacted the nurse supervisor, who inspected both the patient's medication list and the transcribed one, and caught the transcription error before any harm occurred.[1]

> *"Lucky patients will have a family member or close friend who can rise to the occasion. But for most of us, a professional advocate is vital for those situations."*

✚ Patients or their advocates should verify the accuracy of the medication reconciliation lists after they have been transcribed. You'll need to ask sensitively, e.g., "Could I review that list with you?"

IN THE MOMENT: WHAT TO DO

Recall Myra's story about her mother's care from Chapter 5. Myra had sensed that something was missing from the care her mother was getting in the hospital. Myra remained polite while being assertive with the nurses, who ultimately provided her mother the intravenous fluids she'd lacked, rapidly restoring her. Myra was sensitive, persistent and assertive in the hours after the error was made, even though she was uncertain of the truth, and anxious about her mother's health. Ernest Hemingway famously defined courage as "grace under pressure."[2] That's the kind of courage that patient advocates need in the moment. That's rare. Lucky patients will have a family member or close friend who can rise to the occasion. But for most of us, a professional advocate is vital for those situations.

During crises, it is important to rally special attention both from the hospital's clinicians and from your own network of a family member and/or professional advocate. By acting promptly you can reduce the harm of many errors. For example, if you notice that a nurse has given the patient an overdose of a drug, by intervening promptly you can ensure a nurse doesn't give the same overdose the next day.

You should start by asking a member of your clinical team, like Myra did. But you don't have to stop there, and you shouldn't. The nurse or doctor who made the mistake may well minimize its importance, or confidently brush off your questions. That's common distasteful human behavior when someone feels embarrassed, threatened, shamed, scared – or overconfident. Twenty years ago, when I asked the young resident the meaning of the rhythmic spikes on the graph of my pregnant wife's abdominal contractions, she confidently dismissed them as normal and nothing to worry about. I believed her and didn't ask why the peaks recurred consistently. The reason: she was in labor, which her doctors didn't realize until the next morning. The moral of the story: Someone who makes you feel stupid or gives you an answer you don't understand is not your partner.

✚ **Insist on getting a responsive answer that you understand.**

Of course, you'll need them on your side. But you won't know if their incompetence caused the error, or if the hospital's systems caused the error. If it was their incompetence, you'll want other clinicians on your team. And if the hospital's systems caused the error, you'll need other insiders on your team.

Consider multiple errors, when a patient experiences the same error more than once. These occur all too often, abetted by a hospital's automated drug dispensing machines (imagine vending machines with medications in place of candy and soda). If a pharmacy technician stocks the wrong medication in the drawer of such a machine, a nurse who withdraws a drug from that drawer is likely to give that wrong drug to the patient consistently throughout his hospital stay, and, indeed, to other patients. That caused the death of three babies in an Indiana hospital in 2006.[3] A similar mix-up led to the administration of near-fatal thousand-fold overdoses of heparin to actor Dennis Quaid's twins.[4] They were given adult doses of heparin, a powerful blood thinner. If you merely brought the mistake to the attention of the nurse, she might be more mindful of giving the right drug next time – but she might not think of and remove the source of the problem, e,g., the incorrect stocking of the drug dispensing machine. If not, the nurse on the next shift might well commit the same error. To prevent that you need to get the attention of someone in the hospital who is responsible for the safety of the systems the hospital is using. This can be the hospital's patient advocate or risk manager, who would consider, and promptly remedy, the source of the problem, preventing future similar errors.

The goal of asking the risk manager or the hospital's own patient advocate to get involved is to get you especially vigilant care throughout the rest of the hospital stay. That can take different forms. Most errors are set up by the hospital's standard operating procedures rather than by the incompetence or carelessness of staff. So the fact that one clinician made an error affecting you probably doesn't mean you should have them dismissed from your care team. If you trust the clinician who committed the error, you should say so to them and to the risk manager, and ask that they be kept on the clinical team. Hard proof of their competence will be lacking at the time you need to make the decision, so you'll need to rely on your intuition.

When my father was in hospice, gravely ill with Parkinson's disease, I noticed that the hospice nurse had missed a dose of my father's Sinemet, the main drug he took to control his tremors. I asked her about it, and she said he didn't need it. I trusted her and didn't dispute it. Perhaps she had decided consciously to withhold the drug, or perhaps it was a rationalization of her failure to follow a doctor's order. In any event, my intuition had to be my guide. In hindsight, the decision was a good one, as my father remained free of further tremors and continued to receive her compassionate and competent care through the end of his life.

If, on the other hand, after the nurse or doctor learns of their error and you suspect they will act carelessly or incompetently again, fire them from your care team. To do so, write, sign and date that request in a note to the risk manager and ask in the note that it be added to the patient's medical record.

Either way, you should notify the risk manager that you are aware that an error occurred. Your request of the risk manager is important for two reasons. First is to get additional clinicians' attention, e.g., as they provide for VIP care. Second is to have the risk manager identify the systems that likely set up the error and prevent them from repeating an error. For example, assume that the incorrect stocking of an automated drug dispensing system had set up the error. In investigating the matter, the risk manager would learn that and would ensure that pharmacy technicians correctly restocked the medications, preventing future errors. The risk manager will almost certainly speak to the nurse or pharmacist to educate them (via "in-service training") not to do it again. That by itself would not make the medication system any safer for long, so you shouldn't be satisfied if that is the only remedy the risk manager mentions.

You should describe the error in writing to the risk manager, and to add that if a second error occurs, no matter what the cause, you will have the patient transferred promptly to another hospital. That tells the risk manager that you are an empowered patient who will not be satisfied with the usual, nearly useless assurances that the guilty will be retrained.

THE MONTH AFTER

If the results of a medical procedure or treatment are not what you expected, you should ask for a clear explanation. It's likely that the provider will not give you an explanation in writing, though you can try contacting them by email, and perhaps they will reply. You might be more likely to learn something by calling them on the phone. A face-to-face meeting may not be very productive because a lawyer will probably attend, and if so will warn the provider not to say anything that could open the door for a lawsuit. The act of apologizing itself could show responsibility, and providers will rarely apologize. This refusal to apologize or take responsibility for their error is infuriating to surviving family members, and yet it is quite common. This is one of the largest gaping wounds in the patient-provider relationship.

If you have reached a dead end in your efforts to get doctors and nurses to admit their error or apologize, you can try this: Offer, in writing, to formally waive your right to sue in exchange for a full explanation by an involved doctor or nurse and a commitment to create a lasting safeguard, not dependent on the memories of clinicians, to prevent the same error from recurring.

More elaborately, Kathleen Clark, the founder and CEO of Servant Lawyership in Pleasant Hill, Calif., uses such an innovative approach, as she describes:

> *My dearest friend lost her son to medical error in 2003. She and her family did not receive a call, a letter or a visit from the provider. I suggested a letter to the provider from me as their advocate, not their attorney. They eventually got an attorney and later resolved their case for substantial damages. I wrote on their behalf asking for a meeting, a conversation, an opportunity for the family to ask questions, a chance for the family to describe their firsthand observations of the healthcare their son received, and their suggestions for improvement. I told the providers that I knew they had the best of intentions, had compassion for their patients, wanted to help, and wanted the best for the family.*
>
> *It took three letters to get a response. By the time I got a response and the providers were willing to meet with the family, the litigation had settled. Because settlement had already occurred, it was clear that the providers were not agreeing to meet with the family to save money or to settle the case under a confidentiality agreement (while admitting nothing). Both individuals who left me messages about meeting with the family mentioned the tone of my letter, such that they immediately responded to my proposal.*

> *The result was several meetings between my friend and the provider to discuss her son's treatment. She was invited to tell her son's story to 25 urgent care physicians, which she did. The provider made several substantial changes in its system based on her many suggestions and observations. As a result, she and her husband and surviving son still get their healthcare through this provider.*[5]

Whether or not you pursue such an approach, you are free to contact the state Department of Public Health, which will formally investigate serious errors. The state's Board of Registration in Medicine will consider serious errors by doctors, and you can contact them, too, as appropriate. You can contact the Joint Commission on Accreditation of Healthcare Organizations (JCAHO) and urge them to ensure the hospital has a safeguard in place and has performed a root cause analysis of the error at their next formal review of the hospital. You can send a certified letter to the hospital CEO each time you write to one of these organizations, e.g., one week apart, with a copy of the letter, asking for a meeting. Follow up with a phone call, and repeat as needed. You can bring a patient advocate to the meeting to help you learn what happened.

"This refusal to apologize or take responsibility for their error is infuriating to surviving family members, and yet it is quite common."

Medicare patients experiencing an error should file a formal complaint with the Medicare Quality Improvement Organization in their state. QIOs are a resource for Medicare beneficiary complaints about the quality of hospital care. Now, thanks to a policy stimulated by a lawsuit filed by Alan Levine (whose story appears in Chapter 11), you will be able to learn the results of their investigation.[6]

It's important to ask for a safeguard that doesn't rely on memory. Typically the corrective response to an error is to tell staff what happened and hope they remember not to do that again. But relying on memory is a weak safeguard because the pace of medical care is so often so fast. And staff are often tired, interrupted or careless. Sooner or later they'll forget again, with tragic consequences.

A tragic case in point occurred with a would-be hospital client. (In my organizational consulting practice, I advise hospitals on preventing medical errors.) A few years earlier, the death of a patient had triggered a visit from the Department of Public Health. The hospital's chief of nursing recalled that the DPH inspector "tore me a new asshole." The hospital promised to take corrective action, and trained staff not to commit that kind of error again. A few years later, the exact error happened again, resulting in a young girl's death. The hospital staff had forgotten the lesson. Dreading the outcome of another visit from the DPH inspector, the chief of nursing called me in to help. They arranged for me to meet with the CEO, their legal counsel, and the chief nursing officer. I urged them to apologize to the parents, but the lawyer's advice that the CEO and hospital staff stay quiet trumped mine.

✚ Ask that the error be formally reported within the hospital to the risk manager. You can write to the risk manager and verify the error has been reported. You can also ask that the case be presented to the hospital's next morbidity and mortality meeting, where staff will discuss the error and the best response to it. Write that request in a certified letter, and ask the risk manager to inform you in writing of the decision of whether the meeting will consider your case. Even if "in-service training" of staff is the only safeguard they adopt, it's better than nothing.

THE MONTH AFTER THAT

A family member of the immediate victim of the error can suffer too. Tricia Pil, MD, a pediatrician, medical writer and patient advocate living in Pittsburgh, refers to the trauma she experienced in the birth of her son:

> *It took me a year after my son's birth before I was able to verbalize what had happened to me, and even then it was only in a letter to the hospital and physicians involved in our care. It then took another year before I found the Medically Induced Trauma Support Services (MITSS) group while surfing the Web one night and decided to call their 800 number. I will never forget MITSS CEO Linda Kenney personally taking my call late on a Saturday night. It was only after I hung up that I realized that I had just spent two hours pouring out all my grief, pain and anger to a complete stranger over the phone. There are tears in my eyes even as I'm writing this. I really can't overstate what a gift it was that*

> *she gave me that night, just to know that I was not the only one, which is very empowering.*
>
> *Patients who have experienced medical trauma often want to connect with others who have also had personal experience with medical error and adverse events, and that's another step in the process of recovery where advocates can help. Because many have been through it themselves and know firsthand the frustrations of dealing with various players involved in an adverse or unexpected medical event, professional patient advocates can be a particularly valuable resource for patients and families. Finally, for patients who have reached a point where they are seeking to turn their personal negative experience into a transformative force for change and improvement, advocates can serve as mentors and colleagues.*[7]

Most family members of medical error victims lack that vital support. Worse, the system often adds insult to the injury in an appalling way. For an historical parallel, look back to China's Great Leap Forward, when avid revolutionary Maoists committed some particularly awful actions. After executing enemies of the revolution, they were said to collect money from surviving family members for the cost of the bullets that had been used.[8] In American healthcare, just as repellently, in paying providers for services rendered, we, or our insurers, often pay for actions that caused injury or death.

A study by my esteemed colleague Dr. David Bates revealed that one in 10 patients had serious preventable drug errors during their treatment at six selected community hospitals in Massachusetts.[9] Patients pay for these errors, as hospitals routinely bill the health insurers. The insurers pay and then build in all their costs when they set our insurance premiums and send the bill to our employers and us. The most powerful thing we can do as patients is to urge our insurers not to pay for hospital errors that we suffer. Insurers could withhold payment to the hospital, which would send the hospital the right message. Otherwise, given the reimbursement system, hospitals could benefit financially for additional days of hospital care that were incurred because of an error. (This sounds insane, and it is, as I know all too well from my work in patient safety.) Consumers must demand safer hospital care. Strangely, this could be the best way to get it.

Some of the largest insurers think so, too. Medicare, and now Blue Cross Blue Shield and some other insurance companies, have adopted a formal policy to withhold payment for certain very rare events that should never occur ("never events"):

- Wrong surgeries (wrong patient, wrong body part or wrong procedure).
- Deep bedsores ("pressure ulcers of Stage III or IV").
- Catheter (tube)-associated urinary tract infections.
- Blood vessel ("vascular") catheter-associated infections.
- Surgical site infection in the mid-chest ("mediastinitis") following a coronary artery bypass graft (CABG).
- Air embolism (an internal mass of moving air bubbles).
- Blood incompatibility.
- Foreign object retained after surgery.
- Falls and trauma.
- Surgical-site infections following certain orthopedic procedures, or following bariatric surgery for obesity.
- Manifestations of poor blood sugar ("glycemic") control.
- Deep vein blood clot ("thrombosis", or DVT) or a blood clot in the lung ("pulmonary embolism") following certain orthopedic procedures.[10]

Months after such an error, after the shock and horror have faded, you can contact the insurer to make sure that the hospital and physician did not profit from the error. To do so, you can send an email message or letter to the member services unit of your insurer, directing them to withhold payment. If you don't do that, it is very likely that the insurer will routinely pay the hospital and physician, because the insurer will rarely know from the electronic claim they receive that such an error occurred. Your letter will prompt some questioning by the hospital's financial staff of the clinicians. These questions may lead the clinicians to consider, and to learn, what happened. Ideally the hospital will formally investigate it and create some safeguard to save other patients from such an experience.

This is particularly important because this may be the first time that those doctors or nurses, and particularly their superiors who can remedy the system, will learn of the error, for many reasons. Perhaps the doctors or nurses were ashamed. Perhaps no one wants to risk a surgeon's wrath, for example, by telling him. Probably no one has formal responsibility for notifying the surgeon of the error. The consequences may only appear days later. As a result, only 5 percent of injurious medication errors ("adverse drug events") are ever formally reported, and it is common for surviving family members to say that they never received any formal acknowledgment, nor even any hint, from anyone in the hospital that they had blundered.[11] Even if an error is known to hospital staff, two devilish financial incentives play a role in silencing the discussion that improvement efforts require. Hospitals make money from readmitted patients. Second, surgeons bring in revenue to the hospital, and hospitals don't want to anger their golden geese. In short, shame, lack of responsibility for reporting errors, fear of reporting them, and the fear of financial loss minimize the learning that could come from errors and block the development of safeguards.

You, as a survivor, have the power to pierce that, if you choose, and to save someone else's loved one by telling your story, exploring a lawsuit, or changing the law. For many people, the initial rage leads them to consider a lawsuit. To investigate that, begin by contacting a lawyer. A lawyer friend might help, as for Sharon, described later in Chapter 9. She won a modest out-of-court settlement. You can ask your state's Bar association to recommend several medical malpractice lawyers.

If you suffered from a medical device, or a medication, you may be able to join a class action suit. In a class action suit, each victim pays only a small amount to a law firm that acts on behalf of everyone who is affected in the same way. By collecting a small amount from a large number of victims, the law firm can afford to mount a well-financed case. This is important because many device manufacturers and pharmaceutical companies are very large and pay for large legal departments that will probably otherwise vastly outgun you.

For example, the 27,000 plaintiffs who had taken the drug Vioxx formed such a class and eventually each won awards, after attorneys' fees, of $72,000. They had taken Vioxx for a month or more and had a heart attack or stroke within two weeks of taking the drug. The payouts for such harm are quite small but are far from negligible. The overall amount paid by Merck, the maker of

Vioxx, exceeds $3 billion, hopefully a cost large enough to encourage more diligent review by Merck of the safety of their next new drug.[12]

➕ To find out about relevant class actions, look on the Internet, e.g., on Google, searching for web pages with both the phrase "class action lawsuit" and your issue.

Sometimes it is a rude surprise to learn that you cannot file a lawsuit, for any of several reasons. Mary Hight had moved into a nursing home in her late 80s, and was diagnosed a year later, in 2003, with congestive heart failure. The next year, when she became very dehydrated and fell ill for days, her nursing home refused to call an ambulance, despite the urging of Mary's daughter, Janice. Instead, Janice had to push her mother in her wheelchair to the emergency room herself. Mary Hight died there the next day from heart failure. The family was surprised to learn that their contract with the nursing home required binding arbitration to settle disputes. The arbitrator found the nursing home had been negligent but refused to award punitive damages. The settlement went entirely to the family's lawyers, and Mary's son said, "We didn't get one cent." Nursing homes often write in such requirements into their contracts to limit their potential losses.[13]

➕ Question nursing home admissions personnel closely. If an arbitration agreement is mandatory, write on the contract that you're being given no choice. Write, "I'm signing this because I was told I have to."

If you are not able to file a lawsuit, or choose not to, you can and should choose to tell your story. My blog – PatientSafetyBlog.com – consists of the stories of hundreds of people's encounters with the healthcare system. You can contribute your story to warn others and teach them the lessons you learned the hard way.

Demian McElhinny learned through the painful experience of his botched spinal surgery, which has left him impoverished. Demian is a former pharmacy technician for a hospice in Texas, and in his mid-thirties is the father of two boys. His neurosurgeon later admitted to the Texas Medical Board that he was addicted to a narcotic cough syrup and had written fraudulent prescriptions. However, Texas voters had limited malpractice awards four years before Demian's injury, and he emerged afterwards with only "pennies on the dollar" of the settlement he sought.

He writes, "It is atrocious that these doctors do not carry enough liability insurance. Not to mention that the Texas Medical Board did not pull his license; barely reprimanding the doctor at all. Who is out there to protect the patient from these doctors? Something needs to be done. These doctors need to start taking responsibility for their actions and the Texas Medical Board needs to start doing what they are supposed to be there to do...protect the community."[14]

> To see if arbitration or state laws limit your right to sue, you may need to consult a lawyer. Contact your state's Bar Association to find a nearby lawyer who specializes in your issue area.

IN THE LONG RUN

A serious medical error divides your world into the time before it and ever after. For the survivors it may feel that nothing will ever be the same again, much as some people felt after the awful tragedy of September 11, 2001. Life is entirely different, and yet as one medical error survivor says, you can ultimately be happy again.

A faulty water heater in the family's new home badly burned 18-month-old Josie King in January 2001. She recovered quickly at a renowned academic medical center. But just before she was about to be sent home, she received a shot of methadone, which on top of dehydration and an undiagnosed central line infection, was too much for her. She had a fatal cardiac arrest.

Josie's family, particularly her mother, Sorrel King, was devastated. She saw a grief therapist, who worked at a hospice. She spoke on the phone with other women who had survived similar shocks, joining a sisterhood of fellow mourners. She began writing her thoughts as a way to voice them, and ultimately release them. She began to practice the guitar as a distraction. For a time, she found reading books helpful. She tried reconnecting with her religion through a minister and a church group, but this didn't feel helpful.

The medical center offered to pay a settlement. After weeks of consideration, the Kings accepted the payment. Not long after that, Sorrel's therapist challenged her to use her anger to create something positive. Sorrel and her husband Tony launched the Josie King Foundation. They looked for an in-house physician at the medical center who could be their partner and were referred to Dr. Peter Pronovost. That began a long fruitful partnership between Sorrel and Dr. Pronovost, whose father had died from a medical error long before, as told in Chapter 2.

The two formed the Josie King Pediatric Patient Safety Programs at the medical center. The Kings gave much of their settlement payment back to the medical center to finance the programs. The money was earmarked for the two patient floors where Josie had received treatment. Sorrel's generosity was remarkable, especially because she still felt no sense of forgiveness. Indeed, that was one reason that her involvement with the church had been so unsatisfying: the minister's plea that she forgive the people at the medical center felt horribly wrong at that time. Much later, she received a long, heart-felt handwritten letter from the anesthesiologist explaining what happened and why. That was a turning point; only then was she able to forgive the hospital staff.

Dr. Pronovost arranged for Sorrel to speak at a conference of the Institute for Healthcare Improvement, the preeminent organization for improving the quality of healthcare. A segment on the TV show *Good Morning America* soon followed. So did a baby boy.

Since then, Sorrel has conceived a series of projects and resources, five of which are described in her book, *Josie's Story*. The Patient Safety Group provided a Web-based project management tool by which hospitals could share their patient safety issues and efforts with others. The Care for the Caregiver Program treats the second victim of medical errors – the clinician. Removing Insult from Injury trains doctors, nurses and other caregivers in what to say after a medical error. Family Initiated Rapid Response Teams, described earlier in this book, were her baby. Care Journals for Patients are notebooks, now available as a free iPhone app, in which family members record all the details about inpatient hospital stays.

Patient advocate leaders often don't learn about the positive effects of their work. Patients who remain alive because of safer hospital systems rarely realize that a specific safeguard saved them. So it was particularly gratifying for Sorrel to learn that her work had had substantial impact among Michigan hospitals working with Dr. Pronovost. In the Keystone ICU project, 127 teams formed a coalition to eliminate medical errors in the state's intensive care units. They used Josie King's story to inspire them. At the wrap-up conference, Sorrel learned that the hospitals had almost halved central-line infections. After reading the thankful notes written by many of the team leaders, and hearing that this effort had saved the lives of more than 1,500 people, she realized that her devastating loss and her impassioned efforts afterward had ultimately led to the rescue of many other people. This seems to have been a major milestone in her return, years after Josie's death, to happiness.[15]

We'll never know who Josie would have become, had she lived. We have more of a sense of who Lewis Blackman might have become, had he lived. By age 15, Lewis had already acted with the South Carolina Shakespeare Company. At age 15 he took the preliminary college board exam and received the highest score recorded among ninth graders that year at his private school.

Lewis entered an academic medical center in 2000 for an elective surgical procedure to insert a metal strut to support his breastbone. He and his family had hoped it would prevent future respiratory problems from the sunken chest ("pectus excavatum") he had been born with. But the painkilling drug Toradol he received after the operation caused a perforated ulcer. Hospital staff told his mother, Helen Haskell, that constipation was causing his severe abdominal pain. Staff refused to get help despite Helen's repeated requests, nor did they perform a routine blood test that would have flagged the bleeding. A cardiac arrest, and Lewis Blackman's death, followed.

His parents had an autopsy performed, which helped them determine the roles that Toradol and the staff's errors had played. Over the next year and a half, his mother met with hospital staff three times on her own initiative. She also hired a lawyer, who negotiated a settlement with the hospital without the need to go to court. With the money, Helen set up a foundation and started a patient safety advocacy organization – Mothers Against Medical Error (MAME).

By 2005, she had persuaded state legislators in South Carolina to pass the Lewis Blackman Hospital Patient Safety Act. This requires the identification of clinicians and their role in treatment, that hospital patients be given a means of contacting their doctors directly, and that emergency medical help be promptly accessible to patients when needed for urgent patient care concerns. The following year, the South Carolina Hospital Infection Disclosure Act became law, with her help as one of many supporters. In 2007, the Medical University of South Carolina established and funded a lifetime position for a medical school professor via the endowed Lewis Blackman Chair of Clinical Effectiveness and Patient Safety.

Early 2008 saw the creation of the Lewis Blackman Patient Safety Champion Awards Program, sponsored by MAME along with Health Sciences South Carolina, South Carolina Hospital Association (SCHA), and PHT Services Ltd., to commend people who demonstrate exemplary dedication and leadership in advancing the quality and safety of healthcare for patients across South Carolina. Later that year, the Medical University of South Carolina (MUSC) opened the state-of-the-art Health Care Simulation Center for advanced instruction of doctors and nurses.[16] In more mundane work in between these major milestones, Helen sends frequent email messages with news on patient safety to her extensive network.

Other patient safety heroes have also come to the field after the death of loved ones. John James wrote *A Sea of Broken Hearts* about the medical errors leading to the death of his athletic 20-year-old son John. The elder John also regularly writes an e-newsletter, *Patient Safety America*, to educate readers on patient safety.[17]

Michael Rowe wrote movingly of his late son Jesse's two liver transplants and the related medical misadventures in *The Book of Jesse*, which is also an elegy that lovingly describes the artistic teenager.[18] Rowe is a sociologist at Yale University. Following Jesse's death, he has broadened his research focus to include the psychology of medical errors.

The work of the patient safety leaders may well have helped them heal after their traumas, but they have paid an awful price. As Rabbi Harold Kushner said about the wisdom he had gained from his son Adam's suffering from the terminal condition of progeria, he would give it all up in a minute if it would bring back his son.[19]

IF THE WORST HAPPENS

An autopsy played a pivotal role in safeguarding huge numbers of people from one drug's harmful side effect. Millie Beik's son, John Eric Kauffman, died in his 40s. She insisted on an autopsy, which revealed that her son had died from an irregular heartbeat. In taking the drug Zyprexa for six years, his blood pressure had risen, causing his heart to become enlarged from the extra load and causing the irregular heartbeat. Rather than suing the drug maker, Millie told her story to the *New York Times*. The *Times* published a series of stories on the front page, warning millions of its readers about the dangers of Zyprexa.[20]

> ✚ If your loved one has died unexpectedly in the hospital, ask the doctor and nurse for an autopsy to save others from the same fate.

Sorrel, Helen, John, Michael, and many other patient safety leaders started by trying to prevent the recurrence of the errors that claimed the lives of their children. As time went by, the effects of their work have rippled outward to prevent other kinds of errors. Sorrel and Helen, for example, have aggressively promoted the use of rapid response methods to proactively rescue deteriorating hospital patients. While they may feel more energized on some days than others, their commitment seems as permanent as a mother's love.

A PROFESSIONAL PATIENT ADVOCATE CAN HELP YOU:

- Decide whether to transfer your family member to another hospital.
- Decide whether to sue.
- Decide how to ask to be made whole.
- Get an explanation or apology from medical providers.
- Safeguard that provider's standard operating procedures to keep others safe in the future.

1. Interview with Tammy Alvarez, Dec. 5, 2010, Orlando.
2. Ernest Hemingway, New Yorker magazine, Nov. 30, 1929.
3. Deanna Martin, "Two preemies die in Indiana after overdoses," Seattle Post Intelligencer, September 18, 2006.
4. Tara Parker-Pope, "A Hollywood Family Takes on Medical Mistakes," NY Times, March 17, 2008.
5. Email communications with Kathleen Clark, November 2010.
6. Office of Inspector General, "Memorandum Report: Quality Improvement Organizations' Final Responses to Beneficiaries' Complaints," OEI-01-09-00620, September 2010.
7. Email communications with Trisha Pil, November 2010.
8. Harrison Salisbury, China: 100 years of revolution, New York: Holt, Rinehart, and Winston, c1983.
9. Nick King, editor, "Saving Lives, Saving Money: The Imperative for Computerized Physician Order Entry in Massachusetts Hospitals," released by the Massachusetts Technology Collaborative (MTC) and the New England Healthcare Institute (NEHI), Feb. 14, 2008.
10. National Quality Forum, "Serious Reportable Events (SREs): Transparency, accountability critical to reducing medical errors and harm" Fact Sheet at www.qualityforum.org/Publications/2008/10/Serious_Reportable_Events.aspx
11. Cullen DJ, Bates DW, Small SD, et al. "The incident reporting system does not detect adverse drug events: a problem for quality improvement." Jt Comm J Qual Improv 1995; 21: 541-548.
12. Alex Berenson, "Analysts See Merck Victory in Vioxx Deal," NY Times, Nov. 10, 2007.
13. Nathan Koppel, "Nursing Homes, in Bid to Cut Costs, Prod Patients to Forgo Lawsuits," Wall St. Journal, April 11, 2008, pages A1 and A14.
14. Ralph Blumenthal, "After Texas Caps Malpractice Awards, Doctors Rush to Practice There," New York Times, Oct. 5, 2007; private email communications from Demian McElhinny, Oct. 23, 2007 and Oct. 24, 2007.
15. Sorrel King, Josie's Story: A Mother's Inspiring Crusade to Make Medical Care Safer, NY: Atlantic Monthly Press, 2009. The foundation maintains a website, www.josieking.org, that provides patients, families and healthcare professionals with patient safety updates and the latest news on these and new projects.
16. Jill Coley, "Simulation center has lifesaving goal," Charleston Post and Courier, June 12, 2008; Email correspondence with Helen Haskell, July 3, 2007; and Max Alexander, "Night Shift Nightmare," Reader's Digest, June 2007, at www.rd.com/content/night-shift-nightmare/
17. John James, A Sea of Broken Hearts: Patient Rights in a Dangerous, Profit-Driven Health Care System, Bloomington, Indiana: AuthorHouse, 2007.
18. Michael Rowe, The Book of Jesse: A Story of Youth, Illness and Medicine. Washington DC: The Francis Press, 2002.
19. Harold Kushner, When Bad Things Happen to Good People, New York: Schocken Books, 1989.
20. Alex Berenson, "Mother Wonders if Psychosis Drug Helped Kill Son," and "Lilly Settles with 18,000 over Zyprexa," NY Times, January 4 & 5, 2007.

CHAPTER EIGHT
Coping with Grave Illness

As I came of age during the early 1970s, my father and I greatly appreciated reading Art Buchwald's columns. "I was put on earth to make us laugh," he says in his final book. Buchwald viewed the Alice in Wonderland years of the Watergate scandal as his Camelot, and his droll humor often made us laugh out loud. Buchwald had a long and full life, and developed kidney disease ("end stage renal disease") late in life. He chose hospice care, which left him free to be at home rather than on dialysis. As he put it in a column after a year-long curtain call, "it sounded like the most painless way to go, and you don't have to take a lot of stuff with you…I'd like to think some of my printed works will persevere – at least for three years – [maybe] I will wind up on a cereal box top."

Motherless from birth, Buchwald thrived on the love he received from friends while in the hospice. He was able to eat whatever he wanted and do what he pleased. Indeed, he lived far longer than anyone had expected. He had time to recruit friends and family to write eulogies to be published in his final book. There, his daughter wrote, "It's such a joy to see Dad so content. He came to terms with his own death, which most of us never get a chance to do."[1]

They say, he who laughs last, laughs best. If you listen closely, you can hear Buchwald's gales of laughter from the grave.

This chapter is divided into two parts: what you can do, and your ill family member can do, in advance; and what to do when you need to decide on behalf of a gravely ill family member.

> *"My father resolved that he did not want to live as long as she had in such a condition and wrote an advance directive."*

IN ADVANCE

Buchwald's choice of hospice care enabled him to absorb others' love and feel deep contentment, which gave his family the same feeling. Instead of remembering him on dialysis, they remember him as he exited laughing. He became a poster child for hospice care, teaching others through his final interviews, his columns and his own example.

My father had also thought ahead about how best to spend his final time. His mother had been the matriarch of the family, who had arrived in the U.S. from Eastern Europe as a teenager with her father. She had a long life in New York City and eventually developed severe Alzheimers' disease, which progressed through her 80s. I remember my father coming home from visiting her, deeply shaken that she had not recognized him, her only son. My father resolved that he did not want to live as long as she had in such a condition and wrote an advance directive.

He provided copies to my mother and his three adult children. So, late in life, when he himself developed dementia from Parkinson's disease, we knew his wishes, even though he could no longer describe them coherently. He didn't want to try a pallidotomy (a form of brain surgery), which, in any event, had only ambiguous evidence of effectiveness. Rather, we moved him to hospice care, where he was treated with dignity.

His foresight had set him up to have a comfortable end as he wished, where all his family could say goodbye to him in as natural a setting as possible. He died as he had lived – realistically, unostentatiously, serenely, without drama, egotism or useless commotion.

You should write a living will, also known as an advance directive. If you feel comfortable in naming someone to make decisions on your behalf if you're unable to at that time (as a "health care proxy"), or more formally with other legal powers via a "durable power of attorney," you can do so. You can make this as detailed as you wish. Even a simple advance directive is better than none. The simplest can be, as Dr. John Dykers Jr., describes, a signed and witnessed statement like: "If you can fix me, please do. If you can't fix me, please help me avoid pain, fear, lack of air, hunger, nausea, thirst, loss of dignity, and prolonging the dying process. I understand it might take a few days for you to figure out whether you can fix me or not."[2]

More usefully and elaborately, you can write an advance directive using the Five Wishes format, which elicits your preferences in these areas:

1. Who you want to make health care decisions for you when you can't make them.

2. The kind of medical treatment you want or don't want.

3. How comfortable you want to be.

4. How you want people to treat you.

5. What you want your loved ones to know.

This form is available for a very modest fee from Aging with Dignity. It is legally valid in 42 states.[3]

The term "living will" guides others about what to do for you while you are still alive. There's another way you can offer crucial, unforgettable guidance to loved ones while you're alive, though it's unrelated to improving patient safety. Years ago, while rummaging through our safe deposit box, running across the advance directives for my parents and other family members, the property deeds, mortgage notes, wills, and lists of our assets, I realized that my son and daughter would one day look through them for important information after I died. The documents were all so sober and dry, and so lacking in the spirit of what I most wanted to pass on to them. I realized that the more useful knowledge would be a statement of my love, my guidance, and what I wanted for them. So I wrote letters to them to be opened after my death. (Then I realized, why make them wait until then to read them – and showed them the letters.)

> ✚ With your living will, write letters to your loved ones, and share them while you're alive and healthy.

There was no cure for Buchwald or my father. That, and their expressed preferences, made the treatment/hospice decision clear-cut. Of course, if an effective cure is readily available, the treatment/hospice decision is also fairly clear-cut. A much harder decision arises when the best treatment has little chance of success, and when the patient has not expressed his preferences in advance.

THE TREATMENT/HOSPICE DECISION DURING A HEALTH CRISIS

David Rieff, the son of writer Susan Sontag, faced that difficult dilemma during her long illness. His mother wanted to undergo any treatment, no matter how terrible, that offered a possible cure for her leukemia. Many years before, she had beaten the odds, surviving two bouts of cancer. She had chosen a "Halsted" – a radical surgical operation for breast cancer – developed by the pioneering doctor described in the Introduction. That drastic treatment had worked, feeding her strong sense of optimism. But later, her only hope for remission lay in a bone marrow transplant, which offered a very low success rate. She refused to discuss the possibility of her own death. She had no religious faith that might have made the end easier.

Sontag had done several things right. She had clearly told her doctor her preferences, which were to do everything possible to save her life. She was true to her spirit: she was willful, hopeful and avid throughout her life, and always felt that she was exceptional, that the normal odds didn't apply to her. But her avoidance of thinking about death and telling her son how best to help her hope and cope in her final days caused him lasting pain.

"A much harder decision arises when the best treatment has little chance of success, and when the patient has not expressed his preferences in advance."

David did several of the right things: He was with her. He expressed her preferences to doctors when she was unable to. He remained optimistic in talking with her about the future, as she wanted. He disagreed with her choice, in that the bone marrow transplant would lead her to suffer far more physically than if she had chosen pain-relieving ("palliative") care alone. To his credit, David stayed supportive of his mother even though he disagreed with her decision.

Her doctor also acted sensitively in the very difficult situation. Dr. Stephen Nimer told her the prognosis wasn't hopeless. That saved her sanity throughout the illness, though he couldn't save her life. He finessed questions about the odds of survival, while remaining realistic. David says, "In honoring her wishes, without for a moment understating the risks, her doctors opted for treating her in the full, human sense of the word." [4]

Sontag lived a remarkable life. But she made her final time harder on her son than it needed to be, leaving him tormented then, and wracked with guilt later, over his choice. She wanted him to lie to her. Her whole life she had worshiped reason, he said, and taught her son that, so her insistence that he remain optimistic put him in a cruel bind.

That prevented him from doing a critical thing. After her bone marrow transplant failed, he could not transform or reframe her hope for living longer into a hope for living well in her remaining days, or into a hope of connecting with her loved ones. In the end, she had a bad death, lacking a sense of closure and closeness with her only son.

We should expect less of doctors. We want them to reverse terminal illness, after they sensitively tell us the precise diagnosis and exactly how little time we have left to live. Doctors don't know how much time a patient will have before death. They know averages and ranges, and they know there's a huge spread among patients' survival times. People age differently. Some people have a strong religious faith or other purpose for living; many do not. Some have a large network of family and friends; others, none. Some have a genetic predisposition to live long lives; others don't.

Doctors know patients may well view any average survival time the doctor tells them as a death sentence. Sontag had become enraged at an oncologist who had been too candid in his pessimism. Perhaps that doctor should have begun his talk by telling them that he tells all patients first and most importantly to live life to the fullest now and to get their affairs in order, regardless of the prognosis.

> When your loved one's daily life and capabilities are no longer anything like the person they truly are, you'll need to face that squarely. You'll feel that you're in a vortex, being spun around by forces beyond your control. It's impossible to stay centered at a time like that. The best thing you can do is to keep asking yourself what your family member would most want, and to consider how that might differ from what you want for them.

Doctors think differently than patients and families. For some of them, saving lives is a calling; for others, it's their job. Either way, since everyone dies in the end, that means they succeed by extending life, by buying time for patients.

Their training, thankfully, reinforces their can-do attitude. So in a crisis, they will act aggressively as rescuers, rather than passively standing by. The reimbursement system pays hospitals to perform procedures, and pays much less for them to house patients without doing much for them. That makes sense in a way. Yet these three forces – doctors' choice of this profession, their training, and hospitals' reimbursement – become counterproductive at the end of life, when truly healthy life is not an option. Then, extending life merely prolongs suffering.

The default treatment in a hospital occurs in the intensive care unit, which some critics call "death by intensive care." Dr. Sam Forman described how this happened to his own mother:

> *My mother, Rose, was a 4'11" firecracker of South Philadelphia womanhood. She fit a disproportionate interest in humanity and a high decibel level into a small package. That came in handy when she worked during World War II as an inside riveter in the nether regions of B-24 Liberator bomber tail sections: she was a real-life Rosie the Riveter.*
>
> *Much later, in her 80s, she was struck by a heart attack. Over the course of a year, she became the consumer of a dizzying array of specialist physicians and nurses, high-tech diagnostics, cardiac surgery, novel pharmaceuticals, therapeutic devices, and specialty-care facilities. As the family member most suited to be her guide through the maze, I was struck by the providers of all stripes poised with hair triggers to unleash the most novel, the most innovative, and coincidentally the most expensive therapies. After initial treatment reversals leading to scant hope of returning to the independent life she treasured, the collective system would not hear the patient Rose's desires for a less aggressive, more personal and dignified approach.*
>
> *After her ordeal finally ended, my siblings and I noted that what Medicare had spent on our mother could have paid for prenatal care in broad swaths of inner-city Philadelphia, or an entire preventive health program in some third-world country. All Rose had wanted was to pass on quietly to, as she viewed it, rejoin her husband, Akiba, who had died 10 years before. All the while, providers, institutions and suppliers were doubtless counting their consumer scorecards. I suspect that the fruitless*

surgical interventions were probably counted as successes, given what I know about the definitions and timeframes of such total quality measures in the increasingly consumer-oriented clinical world. [5]

✚ Remember that you have a choice even if events are proceeding without you. Alternatives to aggressive hospital treatment are available.

"Slow medicine" is one emerging alternative, as Edie Grieg discovered late in life, fearing her very ill husband would have a "death by intensive care." Edie lives at Kendal at Hanover, a retirement community affiliated with Dartmouth Medical School. A nurse practitioner there asked her about the preferences of her 86-year-old husband, Charley, if he was found to have throat cancer, and the trade-offs of the cancer treatment. The nurse deemed it imperative that none of the decision-making be rushed. After taking the time to think it through, Edie decided against the aggressive care that would include biopsies, anesthesia, surgery, radiation, chemotherapy. Charley came back home to the retirement community to die.[6] The geriatrician who practices slow medicine will look with a healthy skepticism at the value of diagnostic tests and will focus more on the preservation of the ability to independently perform the activities of daily life like eating, bathing, toileting, and dressing. [7]

If you don't, you risk experiencing the full armature of the hospital care system. Dr. Bruce Ferrell, the director of the adult palliative care program at a large academic medical center, recalls a patient who got a liver transplant in 2007, developed serious complications, and remained in the hospital for a year. "He had never even been told he would have to live with a ventilator and dialysis. He was never told this was as good as it was going to get." Dr. Ferrell talked with the patient about the possibility of leaving the ICU to go home and receive hospice care. When the surgeon overseeing the patient found out, he furiously said, "We do not use the h-word on my patients! Don't ever come back!" The patient chose to leave.[8]

✚ It's your life, and your choice. For any treatment, ask about the probability of success, its definition, and the likelihood of complications.

The quality of life is more important than its quantity. Consider what final gift you want to give your family: time with you, or time in the hospital? The vast majority of people in Sontag's situation stop fighting and accept the inevitable because of fatigue, fear or the hope of making their final days memorable for those they'll leave behind.[9]

As a family member's advocate, your final views of them will sear themselves into your memory. If they don't have a strong preference, and you need to make the decision, it's better if you see them, in your mind's eye, at peace.

WORKING WITH A PROFESSIONAL PATIENT ADVOCATE:

The advocate can help in either of two cases. If the ill person is lucid, there are two very difficult, nearly contradictory, tasks facing the care team of the healthy family member and doctors. First, they need to tell the ill person the risks and benefits of aggressive treatment and of alternatives. Second, they need to keep hope alive. An experienced professional advocate has the perspective, objectivity and knowledge that will be sorely needed at this time.

Similarly, if the ill person is not lucid, the healthy family member and doctors need to decide on the ill person's behalf, with a clear understanding themselves of the risks, benefits and alternatives. The perspective of a warm, knowledgeable outsider can also be invaluable at this time.

---

1. Art Buchwald, Too Soon to Say Goodbye, NY: Random House, 2006.
2. John Dykers, Jr., Letter to the Editor, Boston Globe, Sept. 9, 2009.
3. Five Wishes: Available through Aging with Dignity at www.agingwithdignity.org/forms/awd_order_form.pdf
4. David Rieff, Swimming in a Sea of Death: A Son's Memoir, NY: Simon and Schuster, 2008.
5. "Would you rather be treated as a patient or a customer?", Q3, a publication of Yale School of Organization and Management, Spring 2008, p. 116.
6. Jane Gross, "For the Elderly, Being Heard About Life's End," NY Times, May 5, 2008.
7. David Loxterkamp, "The Old Duffer's Club," Annals of Family Medicine, Volume 7, Number 3, May/June 2009.
8. Reed Abelson, "Weighing the Medical Costs of End-of-Life Care," NY Times, Dec. 23, 2009.
9. David Rieff, "Miracle Workers?," New York Times Magazine, Feb. 22, 2008.

PART TWO
At Home

CHAPTER NINE

Coping with a Chronic Condition

He had long had problems getting to sleep. In addition to insomnia, he recently had been plagued by a bad cold and suffered from time to time from stage fright. Professionally, though, this hadn't mattered much, and hadn't kept Heath Ledger from having a successful stage career, including an award-winning role as Ennis Del Mar in the movie *Brokeback Mountain*.

He had been taking several prescription drugs. After his shocking death in January 2008, the New York City chief medical examiner found that he had died accidentally from the combined effects of the painkillers oxycodone (the active ingredient in OxyContin) and hydrocodone; two anti-anxiety drugs, Valium (diazepam) and Xanax (alprazolam); Restoril (temazepam) as a sleep aid; and an over-the-counter antihistamine, doxylamine, which is used in decongestants and as a sleep aid. None of the doses had been excessive individually, though their interaction was fatal. The police had found six different medicine bottles in his Manhattan apartment. Three of them had been filled in Europe, where Ledger had recently been filming. That made several physician experts think that different doctors must have prescribed the medicines, as it would be unlikely that one doctor would order them all.

"This is not rock star wretched excess," says Cindy Kuhn, a pharmacology professor at Duke University. "This is a situation that could happen to plenty of people with prescriptions for these kinds of drugs."[1, 2, 3] People with a chronic illness are often taking a large number of different medications."

✚ It's important to get all your prescriptions from a single pharmacy, as most pharmacies have a computer system that will automatically warn of dangerous drug interactions. Ask your pharmacist if her computer has such alerts built into

"Many tests have high rates of false positive results, and you can have them verified by retesting, perhaps with a different test, or at a different laboratory."

it. If not, you can check for interactions of your drugs on the Internet, for free, at a website like www.umm.edu/adam/drug_checker.htm. If you don't feel comfortable doing that, ask your patient advocate to do so.

You can do a wide variety of things to stay safe while living with a chronic condition. This chapter discusses them, from diagnosis to treatment.

IDENTIFYING YOUR LONG-LASTING CONDITION

Matthew Swan kept getting intestinal infections that required frequent visits to the emergency room and prevented him from attending full days of school. "We were told this was just the way it had to be," said his mother. Doctors near his Idaho home told him to eat a high-fiber diet and use laxatives, which hadn't helped. Nor had specialists at a children's hospital in Michigan been able to help.

Matthew's mother researched colorectal programs, spoke to other parents, and chose to go to Cincinnati Children's Hospital. Doctors there realized he had a very rare form of Hirschsprung's disease, a rare congenital condition that limits the ability of the large intestine to process food. They stopped the high-fiber diet and laxatives. They performed surgery and gave Matthew other forms of help to better control his bowel movements. The staff there see part of their job as helping each patient live as normal a life as possible. That means helping people like Matthew to remain continent. Not doing so would be a "glaring deficiency," in the words of Dr. Marc Levitt at CCH.[4]

> ✚ Matthew Swan's mother was unwilling to accept the conclusion that nothing could be done. As a patient advocate, you should research alternative places to get treatment and ask other parents, as she did.

Persistence is vital. Perhaps a special award should go to Sheila Connolly, who was determined to find out the cause of a creeping and crawling sensation that used to keep her awake for hours.

"It took me a long time to find out what it was," she said. "My primary care physician did not know what I had. I was sent to one neurologist who knew what I had but did not know how to treat it [then a second neurologist]. Then I was sent to a third neurologist. This [occurred] over a course of many years."

Sheila, now in her 70s, battled the disorder for 50 years. Restless legs syndrome (RLS) disturbs a person's sleep pattern and is often underdiagnosed and misdiagnosed. With about 12 million people diagnosed with RLS in the U.S. alone, the condition slowly is becoming a more widely recognized condition.

"Some people will get it once a year when they take a long plane ride, some women will get it only just before their period, some people will get it just if they are very tired," said Dr. John Winkelman, Director of Sleep Health Centers at Brigham and Women's Hospital in Boston. "And then there are people who get it predictably, who get it once or twice or four times a week or unfortunately even every night." Doctors don't know exactly what causes RLS, though they know that certain dopamine levels, low brain-iron levels, and a person's genetic make-up are contributing factors.

Medication has helped relieve Sheila's symptoms. Other patients find that changing their daily routines and being aware of their own triggers for it can help. [5]

> ✚ If you feel sure something is wrong, be persistent in looking for a diagnosis. A patient advocate can help you explore your options.

On the other hand, if you have received a diagnosis that you doubt, you can investigate it. Many tests have high rates of false positive results, and you can have them verified by retesting, perhaps with a different test, or at a different laboratory. That would have saved Audrey Serrano from having a nine-year course of treatment for HIV, a terrible disease – that she didn't have. The side effects of the powerful medicines she was prescribed caused depression, chronic fatigue, loss of weight and appetite, and inflammation of the intestine, and she later received $2.5 million from a jury for the misdiagnosis. [6]

> ✚ If you doubt your diagnosis, you may want to schedule additional lab tests to confirm it.

AFTER THE DIAGNOSIS: FINDING THE RIGHT CLINICAL TEAM

People will help you – once you find the right ones for your team. The first and foremost team member is your doctor. The selection of a doctor was discussed in Chapter 1. For people with chronic illness, a doctor's compassion is particularly important. Denise Grady told the story of her sister, who was diagnosed with two forms of cancer at the same time. She needed chemotherapy and radiation, an operation, more chemotherapy, and a smaller operation, all of which consumed a year of her life. The compassion of two doctors played a big part in helping her get through this traumatic time, she later said. The radiation oncologist would sling her arm around her shoulders and walk down the hall as if they were old friends. The medical oncologist closely tracked the side effects of the chemotherapy, suggested remedies, reminded her of the good survival odds, and reassured her that her hair would grow back, as it did. Such supportive physicians greatly help people cope with cancer and less dreaded diseases. [7]

Nurses or paraprofessionals in your doctor's office may be able to help you as well. Many doctors' offices are experimenting with offering a "patient-centered medical home" for their patients. In one of them, for example, Robert Williamson emails and phones his new doctor's office with his heart and diabetes readings. The doctor has hired a patient educator and has acquired supportive technology to monitor patients' treatment and follow-up and remind them of upcoming tests for the early detection of cancer.

"I can get better directions, at the very moment I need them," says Robert, who considers such guidance "life-saving." He contrasted that to the hurried care he got from another doctor, who missed seeing some danger signs that could have prevented or minimized the effects of Robert's subsequent career-ending stroke.[8]

More elaborately, some patients have received devices that gather information while they are at home and send it to the doctor's office electronically. This is known as telemonitoring. Patients with heart disease, for example, use the equipment at home to monitor their heart rate, the oxygen levels in their blood, and their weight. The system in use at Partners Healthcare in Boston asks patients a few questions about how they're feeling, and all the information electronically travels to the home care program's nursing station. So if Mario, an 89-year-old patient living with heart failure in a Boston suburb, gains a pound or two, he gets a prompt phone call from a nurse. That might prevent him from having to enter the hospital yet again.[9]

> ✚ If you have severe chronic illness, ask a professional patient advocate if telemonitoring could help you stay out of the hospital, and if so, to help find the right device for you.

The information the patient gets about self-care via phone, email or telemonitoring represents one of the two main benefits of a patient-centered medical home. The other, ideally, is a sense of accompaniment; in effect, you're home with someone who cares about you. That accompaniment over four years was the key to Maria's recovery, whose story appeared in Chapter 6. Sori patiently encouraged, rather than forced, Maria, to take her medications, to get to her appointments on time, and to renew her Medicaid applications, all of which helped stimulate her long-term recovery.[10] Even in a medical practice that is not funded as a medical home, a nurse may be available to talk with you on a regular basis about how to best keep you in control of your chronic condition.

> ✚ Write a note to your doctor that asks for a nurse to routinely call you to discuss how best to cope with your condition.

Most doctors, though, lack the tracking and reminder systems, telemonitoring, dedicated staff, and incentives to routinely provide these preventive services to all of their chronically ill patients. You should consider hiring a professional patient advocate to either contact you routinely to ensure you stay on course or to help you find that support elsewhere.

MEDICATIONS

The range and power of medications today is remarkable. Of course, they also have the power to cause harm, sometimes severely. Prescription drugs for chronic conditions can interact fatally, as they did for Heath Ledger and Michael Jackson. Accidental overdoses of prescription drugs can also prove fatal. For example, Adam Henderson suffered from chronic hip pain that was a result of a car accident when he was a teenager. To control the pain, he wore a Fentanyl patch on his right arm. Yet the patch leaked, causing a fatal overdose, and he died in December 2003, at age 28. Over the next few years, the U.S. Food and

Drug Administration learned of hundreds of deaths from similar accidents, leading the agency to issue a formal warning in 2007.[11]

More commonly, many other drugs have much less severe side effects. It's always a trade-off; you have to carefully consider the advantages and disadvantages and discuss them with your doctor.

But if some people experience problems in taking too much of a medicine, others take it too little, perhaps because they forget. For these folks, it can be useful to get some kind of device to remind them to take their medicine when the time comes. For example, Harriet Meyers, a Minnesota resident who has kidney disease and takes 10 different medications, uses a medication management system called MedMinder. Basically a computerized pillbox of her medications, the system beeps and flashes when it's time to take one of the drugs. The system sends phone calls and email verification to Harriet's adult children in

> *"Decisions to quit smoking are not made solely by isolated persons, but rather they reflect choices made by groups of people connected to each other both directly and indirectly at up to three degrees of separation."*

New York City and Australia. If Harriet has not taken the medicine at the right time, the system alerts Harriet's daughter promptly so she can call her mother and ask her to take the medicine during the phone call.

Rachel's mother has come to appreciate the device. "At first I was rebellious. I said, 'Look, I'm lining up my pills, Rachel. I know what I'm doing,'" she says. But now she sees it differently: "I decided to try and now I'm hooked."[12]

> ✚ If you're the family advocate for a person who has to take a lot of medicines or has impaired memory, e.g., Alzheimers, you should consider the new systems and technologies to enable them to stay at home safely. A professional patient advocate can help you find an appropriate medication reminder system.

You can learn from others – and teach others – about the effects of the drugs you take. That has been very useful for thousands of people, including Todd Small. Living with multiple sclerosis in Seattle, he would often feel stuck in quicksand. His brain would send an electrical signal meaning "walk," but the signal would snag on scar tissue in the insulating layer of myelin around the nerve, and often it would never reach his foot. For 14 years, Todd had been taking a low dose of baclofen daily. In June 2007, he learned from the website PatientsLikeMe that a higher dose of baclofen was being used safely by 200 others with MS and would not weaken his muscles, as he had been told long ago. He discussed that with his neurologist, who raised the dose. While his foot drop isn't cured, he no longer feels that he's sinking into quicksand when walking to his car. That website collects and aggregates the dosages and experiences of particular groups of patients to enable them to become "co-practitioners" who are treating their conditions with their doctors. [13]

Such websites may also steer you away from drugs that the patient community has found are not helpful for your condition. Karen Felzer, for example, was concerned about her father, who is afflicted with Lou Gehrig's disease (ALS, or amytotrophic lateral sclerosis). Karen's father was taking lithium for the ailment, which didn't seem to be helping. She was able to launch an online study of the use of lithium by these patients. The patients reported lithium was much less effective than a recent Italian study had suggested. Karen's father stopped taking the drug, so he is no longer subjected to its side effects. PatientsLikeMe gathers information for communities of patients with depression and other mood disorders, HIV, Parkinson's disease, Lou Gehrig's disease, and other chronic diseases.[14]

> ✚ Look on websites of online patient communities to learn what other patients with your condition say about the effects of your medications and discuss their conclusions with your doctor. If the online community is hard to find, enlist the help of a patient advocate.

An online patient community also might help you find an experimental drug that could be effective. EmergingMed.com, for example, links cancer patients with clinical trials of new drugs. The service is free to patients and is paid by medical centers and research sponsors. If you or a family member have cancer, you should consider participating in a clinical trial.

> ✚ A professional patient advocate can guide you through the very difficult decision of whether and how to look for a clinical trial, and whether to join a specific drug trial.

MORE TEAMMATES: FRIENDS, FAMILY AND COMMUNITY

When you receive a diagnosis of a chronic condition, perhaps the worst thing you can do is retreat into a shell and isolate yourself from others. We are umbilical beings, having received nourishment directly from a mother even before birth. We heal in groups, with a little help from our friends.

Superstar quarterback Tom Brady of the New England Patriots has fully recuperated from his knee surgery in 2008. Yet immediately after the surgery, many Patriots fans were bewildered to see news photographs of their favorite tough guy being spoon-fed and cuddled by his Brazilian supermodel girlfriend. (Showing his trademark gridiron judgment and ability to make smart passes for impressive gains in a crowded field of rivals, Brady later chose to marry Gisele Bundchen.) Experts commented that her touching helped him heal more quickly, and, indeed, that the public demonstration of her touch may have motivated some of his followers to seek the same healing behavior at home. Touching is medicinal, says Dr. Tiffany Field, head of the Touch Research Institute at the University of Miami, and is therapeutic for asthma, cancer and diabetes. Massage and hugging, she says, slow down heart rate and blood pressure and the production of stress hormones.[15]

➕ Hug your personal Gisele, and rub her feet.

You can also be helpful as a friend or relative as an amateur detective and advisor, as Sharon reports her friends were:

> *I had been on Effexor for a good five years at different levels; I had been decreasing it for a long period of time but for years had also been using free samples the doctor had given me. They come in those packs that you push through, and I collected them from other people, so I was happy to have them for free. When I ran out and the drug company stopped sending them, I had to get a prescription and go to the drug store for the first time in a lot of years. I took the script to Sam's. They were great; they handled it. I had it filled and started taking them.*
>
> *I started not feeling well pretty immediately, but I didn't realize that. The next two days, I started not feeling well. My symptoms were nausea and dizziness; I was lightheaded and extremely tired. I had to come home from work about 3:00 to lie down.*

A couple of days later, I called my doctor (not the one who'd prescribed the Effexor) and they fit me in and I went in that day because I'm not usually sick. My friend Joan says I'm always zooming around but saw that I wasn't at all. I started having heart palpitations – that scared me. I went to the doctor's and first he was convinced I was pregnant! He wanted to do a pregnancy test! But I knew I wasn't. I had an EKG and they did a lung X-ray – all these tests! Everything checked out OK, and he basically told me to give it a few more days. It probably was Day 8 now, and I was laying on the couch feeling pretty low. Joan came over, and we were talking about all my symptoms. She asked me all these questions: Have you been eating anything different? Are you taking a new kind of vitamin? Have you changed pharmacies? She said she read an article in Newsweek that the pharmacies made mistakes all the time – she had just read it, and that's how it started. I told her I didn't change pharmacies, and she asked if any of my pills looked different, and I realized they did. But because I'd been getting free samples, I didn't put it together. I was like an idiot – because a lot of times they do.

So the next day, I still took the pill, like an idiot, and I went to the doctor, and I asked him for a copy of the prescription, and I told him what I thought might've happened. The doctor pretty much knew when I told him. So I took the script and the nine pills that I'd taken out of the 30-day prescription, and I took it to the pharmacy, and said, Is this what I am supposed to have here? They said they have a hard copy on their computer files – I didn't know they could do that. And they looked at the script and the bottle, and went, "Woops! This is not what we filled"!

They immediately gave me another bottle of 30 of the right-timed release ones. They told me that they were sorry, and they didn't charge me for the new bottle.

The next day I got a phone call from the pharmacist that prescribed it, apologizing, and wanted to know how I was feeling. The same day, I got a call from an independent insurance agent of some kind, who said that by law they had to report on the error, and she asked me to tell the story of what happened as well. Three days later, I got a call from the same woman, who said that she was able to make me a one-time settlement if I was prepared to accept it today. I said, "What settlement?!" And all this information came out of the blue for me. I told her I was not *willing to make any kind of settlement, that I needed a couple of days to think. She had made me an offer of $1,200.*

I called my friend who is an attorney, and we talked strictly as friends – I wasn't paying him anything. And he explained to me that this could be a huge lawsuit and the company was trying to avoid it, and that I needed to think about how I felt about all of this. I explained to him that I was never thinking about suing, and that I was not comfortable with the idea of getting a lot of money from them. My friend explained to me that I had a legitimate complaint and deserved to be compensated. So we talked about different options as far as my pain and suffering, how much time I missed from work, and all my doctors' bills – I was concerned about that because I work for a nonprofit, for nothing, practically, and I was concerned about all the medical bills I had just created. So we came up with a number that covered all my medical expenses and covered me missing a week of work –$2,200.

Now, I still feel that Sam's has been the best pharmacy for me over the years. They've been great before – and since. Now I always open the bottle of pills when I get there. Mistakes can happen anywhere. It's a business, but it's human beings filling the scripts. It's scary. I tell everybody: Check your meds!

I had two advocate friends. My life is run by my friends. I couldn't make it without my friends.[16]

Friends can help others stop smoking and overeating. "Decisions to quit smoking are not made solely by isolated persons, but rather they reflect choices made by groups of people connected to each other both directly and indirectly at up to three degrees of separation," according to a team of researchers in an article published by the *New England Journal of Medicine*. In other words, the behavior of one's friends, and of the network of their friends, and even the broader community of the friends of the friends' friends, all affect one's likelihood of successfully quitting smoking. The same research team of doctors found a similarly strong effect of social networks on efforts by obese people to lose weight.[17,18]

➕ If you are concerned about a friend, becoming healthier yourself in these ways may well help them get healthier.

If the support of friends and relatives is important in promoting healthy habits, it's also vital if a person is facing cancer. Kerry Herman's husband was able to help his wife make a difficult decision about surgery for her breast cancer. Kerry's mother had had breast cancer at age 49, so Kerry knew she was also at risk. Her yearly mammogram at age 55 showed calcifications, for which a biopsy was recommended. The biopsy revealed very early cancer called ductal carcinoma in situ ("DCIS"). Faced with the removal of her left breast and biopsies of the right one, Kerry consulted her husband. After he said he was more concerned about her health than her breasts, she chose a bilateral mastectomy and breast reconstruction. With the help of her husband, she was able to make a proactive decision. While most women would prefer a different choice, Kerry made her own decision and had the support of her husband in doing so. She feels comfortable with her decision: "I have never regretted my decision. For me, having to go through this every year and wondering if I would beat the Grim Reaper was agony." She notes that a friend with the same biopsy findings chose not to have surgery, ending up with a spreading invasive cancer.[19]

Sometimes a person with cancer doesn't want guidance or any specific form of help. Even then, a friend can be helpful, as they were for Brian Wickman, the manager at a luxury hotel in Manhattan. He had an aggressive tumor in his ankle and later was found to have thyroid cancer. He spent two months in intensive care. His friends called him brave and inspirational. Brian said, "They would put me on a pedestal. That doesn't allow me to be human and in pain, angry or depressed." He would write blunt and sometimes grumpy email messages to friends, adding "This is not a call for pity responses. Just let me be where I am."[20]

➕ Your friend with cancer may want you primarily to be there with him more than he wants your guidance or pity.

As a patient, you may be surprised to find new friends as you grapple with your condition. Through a support group, you may become quite close to others in your situation. Jeffrey Schanz is a case in point. A long-term survivor of glioblastoma, Jeffrey returned to his high-pressure job in the U.S. Department of Justice, and now runs a support group in Washington, D.C. "It's almost unfair to my loved ones," he says, "but I'm more comfortable with brain-tumor survivors because we all know what we've gone through. It's still hard to articulate how hard you have to fight."[21] Cori Liptak, who runs a support group based in Boston's Dana-Farber Cancer Institute for people with brain tumors, says, "These are people who have established friendships outside of Dana-Farber. Once you've seen a patient connect with another patient and be able to say, 'I have a friend who understands,' the power of that type of success goes beyond anything I can really describe."[22]

Beyond the support group's model of healing in groups is an innovative alternative to the standard visit to the doctor. For the vast majority of us, a doctor's appointment is brief and well known: one doctor examines and advises one patient to do something the patient often doesn't want to do. Some innovative doctors arrange a longer appointment with a group of patients. "It was fabulous," said Nicholas Poly, an 80-year-old retired engineer who saw his cardiologist, Dr. Gene Lindsey of Harvard Vanguard Medical Associates in the Boston area, during a 90-minute group visit with eight other patients. "I have problems similar to what other people have. I get to hear their questions, too, and that's good." A study at the Cleveland Clinic found that, when surveyed, many more patients in group appointments called their physician's care "excellent" than did patients in individual appointments. Instead of the physician alone trying to convince a patient to reverse longstanding habits in a rushed individual visit, the more relaxed pace and companionship in group visits ideally allows the group, over time, to create a norm of self-care of the condition.[23]

✚ Ask a professional patient advocate if your local providers offer group visits.

Online communities can do much more than merely provide information on drug treatments. In Chapter 5, LotsaHelpingHands.com was mentioned briefly as a free resource. This was quite helpful to Penny Gordon, a breast cancer survivor in Needham, Mass. A friend, Karen Feltcher, served as the coordinator of services through the website, using its online calendar to schedule help. "People swarmed the website," Karen said. Local friends brought meals and treats, drove Penny to chemotherapy appointments, and car-pooled her kids where they needed to go.[24]

Another broad online community can be found at www.CaringBridge.org. George Lindberg used the website to inform friends and gain support after his diagnosis of stage IV melanoma in a lymph node and adrenal gland. Now, having reached the formal milestone where there is no longer any evidence of his disease, he says, "The uplifting energy I was receiving from my CaringBridge site was at least as valuable to my immune system as any medication I would have taken."[25]

Online communities have also formed for specific conditions for everything from the most common to the most rare diseases. For example, for people with diabetes, Diabetes Mine has become both a community for diabetes patients and an information clearinghouse for helpful treatments and gadgets. For those with certain genetic conditions far more rare than diabetes, a British organization called Unique (at www.rarechromo.org) calls itself on online support group that provides information and support to families and individuals affected by any rare chromosome disorder.

If your friends are Twitter-savvy, they can sometimes provide particularly timely help. Such was the case with Oregon resident Terri Nelson, who had surgery to remove her fibroid tumors. Her investigation of the kind of surgery she should have was described in Chapter 3. Her husband, Stewart Loving-Gibbard, used Twitter, the short-message communication service, to inform friends and family about her surgery and recovery. A friend who received one of the messages responded that Terri's chattering teeth could signal a potentially hazardous side effect ("tardive dyskinesia," i.e., involuntary repetitive movements with a delayed onset) of one of her anti-nausea drugs.[26]

After you've received a diagnosis of a chronic illness, you'll have your work cut out for you. Dr. Mark Beers knows this well and also knows one can take control despite the illness:

I have had diabetes for nearly 45 years. Important factors are within your control. First is your weight. In second place is your diet. And obviously exercise plays a big part of the wellness picture, too. If you are willing to take control, there is very good news indeed: You can avoid the complications of diabetes and lead a healthy life.[27]

YOUR PROFESSIONAL PATIENT ADVOCATE CAN:

- Verify that your medications won't incur drug-drug interactions.

- Help you find a medical practice that feels like a patient-centered medical home.

- Connect you with doctors' practices that can automatically gather information from you while you're at home through telemonitoring.

---

1. Chan, Sewell, "Heath Ledger's Death Is Ruled an Accident," NY Times, Feb. 6, 2008.
2. Associated Press, "Heath Ledger died of accidental overdose," reprinted at http://today.msnbc.msn.com/id/23029566#slice-2 , Feb. 6, 2008.
3. Ledger: James Barron, "Medical Examiner Rules Ledger's Death Accidental," NY Times, Feb. 7, 2008.
4. Swan: Reed Abelson, "Managing Outcomes Helps a Children's Hospital Climb in Renown," NY Times, Sept. 15, 2007, page B1 and B4.
5. Connolly: Paula Rizzo, "Diagnosing Restless Leg Syndrome," Fox News, www.foxnews.com/story/0,2933,296214,00.html , Sept. 9, 2007.
6. Ngowi, Rodrique, "Jury awards $2.5 million to Mass. Woman misdiagnosed with HIV," Boston Globe, Dec. 12, 2007, at www.boston.com/news/local/massachusetts/articles/2007/12/12/jury_awards_25_million_to_mass_woman_misdiagnosed_with_hiv/?rss_id=Boston.com+--+Latest+news
7. Denise Grady, "For Cancer Patients, Empathy Goes a Long Way," NY Times, Jan. 8, 2008.
8. Milt Freudenheim, "Trying to Save by Increasing Doctors' Fees," NY Times, July 21, 2008.
9. See www.connected-health.org video and www.PatientSafetyBlog.com/2008/07/id-land-at-hospital-again-if-not-for.html
10. Behforouz, supra.
11. Kenneth Reid, Adverse Event Reporting News, June 18, 2007, and Lauran Neergaard, Associated Press, Boston Globe, Dec. 22, 2007.
12. Hilary Stout, "Technologies Help Adult Children Monitor Aging Parents Medicine and Health," NY Times, July 29, 2010, page D1 and D7.
13. Thomas Goetz, "Practicing Patients," NY Times Magazine, Mar. 23, 2008, page 32f.
14. Carolyn Johnson, "Through website, patients creating own drug studies," Boston Globe, Nov. 17, 2008, pages B1 and B4, and www.PatientsLikeMe.com .
15. Meredith Goldstein, "Two-hand Touch," Boston Globe, Feb. 11, 2009.
16. Face to face interview, Jan. 2007, Decatur, Georgia.
17. Nicholas Christakis and James Fowler, "The Collective Dynamics of Smoking in a Large Social Network, New England Journal of Medicine, 358;21, May 22, 2008.
18. Nicholas Christakis and James Fowler, "The Spread of Obesity in a Large Social Network over 32 Years," New England Journal of Medicine, 357:4, July 26, 2007.
19. Jane Brody, "Personal Health: For breast health, take the initiative," NY Times, Oct. 21, 2008.
20. Jan Hoffman, "When Thumbs Up Is No Comfort," NY Times, June 1, 2008, Styles section, pages 1, 8-9.]
21. Stephanie Cajigal, "Life after Brain Tumor," Neurology Now, September/October 2008.
22. Cori Liptak (edited by Dawn Stapleton), "First Person," Paths of Progress, Fall/Winter 2008, page 32, published by Dana-Farber Cancer Institute.
23. Liz Kowalczyk, "The Doctor Will See All of You Now," Boston Globe, November 30, 2008.
24. Amy Carboneau, "Community helps woman fight cancer," Needham Times, pages 1 and 17, September 30 – October 6, 2010.
25. At www.caringbridge.org/story_blindberg
26. John Schwartz, "Logging on for a Second (or Third) Opinion," NY Times, Sept. 29, 2008.
27. Mark Beers, Living with Diabetes. AARP/Sterling, 2007.

CHAPTER TEN

Safe Complementary/ Alternative Medicine

She began to practice Ashtanga yoga to get back into shape after the birth of her daughter, Lourdes, in 1996. Madonna has been a devout practitioner of yoga since then, calling it "a workout for your mind, your body and your soul."[1]

You may want proof beyond the testimonial of a cultural icon. There are many devotees of yoga, and to other forms of self-care, for health conditions that are alternative or complementary to conventional medical care. Some articles in the medical literature support the effectiveness of particular forms of complementary/alternative medicine for specific conditions; many more articles are inconclusive, or dismissive. There's a disconnect between the broad use of alternative medicine and the skimpy research base supporting it. That contradiction will be with us for quite some time. In light of that ambiguity, this chapter discusses both sides. The field of complementary and alternative medicine is quite broad, including dozens of kinds of treatments. This chapter considers only a few of the most widely used treatments: acupuncture, faith and prayer, yoga, meditation. Stories of individuals who have used these treatments are accompanied by findings from review articles in the medical literature.

Acupuncture has long been used by Dr. Andrew Weil and far less well-known chronic disease sufferers. Suffering pain in his knee without knowing the cause, Dr. Weil tried acupuncture, rather than cortisone shots or large doses of pain medicine, and felt much better from it.[2]

Many experts have agreed on the effectiveness of acupuncture for certain conditions. After a systematic review of the relevant articles on breast cancer, Dr. Judith Jacobson and her colleagues found that "acupunc-

> *"Many experts have agreed on the effectiveness of acupuncture for certain conditions."*

ture seems to relieve nausea and vomiting associated with chemotherapy."[3] A consensus panel that studied acupuncture for the National Institutes of Health agreed more broadly, concluding that "promising results have emerged showing the efficacy of acupuncture in chemotherapy nausea and vomiting."[4] While acupuncture can be effective for nausea in chemotherapy and chronic low back pain, among others, it is not consistently effective for some other conditions.

> *"If this seems unscientific, it may be that our science has not caught up with ancient wisdom."*

FAITH AND PRAYER

Rabbi Kerry Olitzky describes his family's encounter with his wife's cancer:

> *We don't know where the cancer came from, but during her illness Sheryl taught our family that faith means not to passively accept what life deals you – whatever it is. Rather, we must seize life and struggle with it, using the force of disease against itself, not against the self – which we are prone to do. Physicians do not set the parameters for our struggle. We set the terms, always striving to remain in control, trying not to allow the disease to get the upper hand. This posture is bolstered by faith in ourselves, reflective of faith in God and the covenant we share with the Divine. Faith is the force in the world that makes for healing.*[5]

It's not that one prays to God, who hears, thinks about it, decides favorably, and heals the sick person. Rather, faith sustains the healing life force. If this seems unscientific, it may be that our science has not caught up with ancient wisdom, that our researchers haven't learned to fully observe and prove it yet. Yet there is some substantial supporting evidence for the value of relaxation techniques like prayer and meditation. As Dr. Jacobson noted in another systematic review on treating anxiety and depression among adult cancer patients, the instruction of relaxation skills for newly diagnosed patients produced significant improvement in seven of seven trials on anxiety and six of six trials on depressive symptoms.[6] Various psychosocial techniques were also helpful for cancer patients after they completed medical treatment, according to a study by Dr. Annette Stanton. Her overview of the relevant randomized controlled trials, the gold standard in medical research, found that psychosocial interventions (i.e., those addressed toward physical, psychological and interpersonal challenges) for early-stage breast cancer and prostate cancer patients at re-entry (after medical treatment) can be effective.[7]

YOGA

You don't have to be like Madonna to benefit from yoga. Jim Mielke is about as unlike Madonna as a person can be, a solidly grounded Midwesterner who has long worked in east Asia, far from the limelight, in international development. Jim, a veteran of 11 ostomy surgeries, writes, "The key underlying factors of my coping style that seems to set me apart from the 'fighter' attitude I often hear – 'Joe was always a fighter and wasn't going to let such and such beat him...' – My coping style is distinctly nonconfrontational, going with the flow, and the methods that have helped me are the yoga and meditation."[8] Yoga has also been found to be beneficial for people with depression. In a review article of the most solidly grounded studies, Karen Pilkington and her colleagues reported that all five randomized control trials had found positive effects of yoga for people with depression.[9]

WHEN IN DOUBT

Other complementary and alternative medicine (CAM) treatments may well be effective. A systematic review of studies on relieving cancer patients' pain concluded that "CAM modalities such as hypnosis, imagery, support groups, acupuncture and healing touch seem promising, particularly in the short run," though there are few well designed studies that used randomized control trials.[10]

Another systematic review found, "In the area of cancer symptom management, auricular acupuncture, therapeutic touch, and hypnosis may help to manage cancer pain. Music therapy, massage and hypnosis may have an effect on anxiety, and both acupuncture and massage may have a therapeutic role in cancer fatigue. Acupuncture and selected botanicals may reduce chemotherapy-induced nausea and emesis, and hypnosis and guided imagery may be beneficial in anticipatory nausea and vomiting. Transcendental meditation and the mindfulness-based stress reduction can play a role in the management of depressed mood and anxiety."[11]

An article on the role of exercise for cancer patients that considered all the relevant studies that met a set of quality screens concluded that "cancer patients may benefit from physical exercise both during and after treatment."[12]

Three kinds of findings are common among the review articles. First are the mildly positive findings. Second, the authors note that none of the studies reported any adverse effects. Third, the authors often state that only a small number of well-designed studies have been performed. Given the traditional caution of scientific researchers, the conclusions are hedged and almost lukewarm.

Given that, how should patients and advocates make the decision on using a form of CAM? Most cancer patients use complementary and alternative medicine in hopes of boosting their immune systems, relieving pain, and controlling the side effects of disease or its treatments, rather than in hoping it will cure them.[13] Their use is complementary to conventional medicine rather than a substitute for it.

A different kind of logic is called for. The logic of conventional medicine is to consider whether the benefits of a medication, operation or other treatment outweigh its disadvantages, e.g., the risk of injury or death, side effects and costs. The downsides of today's powerful conventional treatments can be substantial, so to be on the safe side, honoring their professional watchword to do no harm, researchers customarily set a high bar on effectiveness: they agree only to report findings that they are 95 percent certain are due to the treatment, preferably in a randomized control trial. But CAM interventions have little, if any, risk and cost, and are usually complementing rather than substituting for other forms of treatment. Exaggerating to make the point, one can say, if it's free and harmless, even if of uncertain benefit, why not? That's not illogical; it merely sets an appropriately lower bar for using a CAM intervention.

The evidence may be ambiguous because relatively few studies have been funded and performed. There are few TV advertisements for CAM and few lobbyists for CAM on Capitol Hill.

➕ Read about the complementary and alternative techniques to conventional medicine that might help you heal.

A PROFESSIONAL PATIENT ADVOCATE CAN HELP YOU:

- Investigate the consensus among medical researchers on the effectiveness of particular CAM treatments for your condition.

- Help you select CAM treatments that will complement your conventional medical treatment.

- Steer away from CAM treatments that may be harmful.

---

1. Motley Health blog, at www.motleyhealth.com/yoga/madonna-stays-in-shape-with-ashtanga-yoga-workouts
2. Elizabeth Cohen, "5 alternative medicine treatments that work," CNNHealth.com at www.cnn.com/2007/HEALTH/10/04/ep.alt.med/index.html#cnnSTCText , 2009.
3. Judith Jacobson et al, "Research on Complementary/Alternative Medicine for Patients With Breast Cancer: A Review of the Biomedical Literature," Journal of Clinical Oncology, Feb. 2000.
4. NIH "Consensus Development Panel on Acupuncture,"
JAMA, 1998;280:1518-1524.
5. Excerpt by Rabbi Kerry M. Olitzky is from "Facing Cancer as a Family" – part of the LifeLightsT pastoral care booklet series, Jewish Lights Publishing, 2000. Permission granted by Jewish Lights Publishing, Woodstock, VT, www.jewishlights.com.
6. Judith Jacobson et al., "Management of anxiety and depression in adult cancer patients: Toward an evidence-based approach," in Change AE, Ganz PA, Hayes DF, et al (eds.): Oncology: An Evidence-Based Approach, Philadelphia: Springer, 2006, pages 1552-1579.
7. Annette Stanton, "Psychosocial Concerns and Interventions for Cancer Survivors," Journal of Clinical Oncology, Vol. 24, #32, Nov. 10, 2006, pages 1532-1537.
8. James Mielke, email correspondence, Nov. 3, 2007.
9. Karen Pilkington, Graham Kirkwood, Hagen Rampes, Janet Richardson, "Yoga for depression: The research evidence," Journal of Affective Disorders, Vol. 89, Issue 1, pgs 13-24, Dec. 2005.
10. Aditya Bardia et al, "Efficacy of Complementary and Alternative Medicine Therapies in Relieving Cancer Pain: A Systematic Review," Journal of Clinical Oncology, Vol. 24, No. 34, Dec. 1, 2006, pages 5457-5463.
11. Patrick Mansky and Dawn Wallerstedt, "Palliative and Supportive Care: Complementary Medicine in Palliative Care and Cancer Symptom Management," Cancer Journal, September/October 2006 - Volume 12 - Issue 5 - p 425-431.
12. Ruud Knols, Neil K. Aaronson, Daniel Uebelhart, Jaap Fransen, Geert Aufdemkampe, "Review Article: Physical Exercise in Cancer Patients During and After Medical Treatment: A Systematic Review of Randomized and Controlled Clinical Trials," Journal of Clinical Oncology, June 1, 2005, pages 3830-3842.
13. Mansky, Ibid.

CHAPTER ELEVEN

Living for Others

A patient advocate helps other individuals to survive their health crises as comfortably as possible, paving the way for them to thrive afterwards. They work face to face, or by phone, working directly with one client at a time. Some of their colleagues work more broadly to help strangers survive and thrive, whether their actions benefit a single person or many of them at once. This chapter explores those efforts, starting with the broader successes, before discussing smaller, more conveniently accomplished kindnesses to strangers.

In December 2010 I received the best Chanukah gifts of my life: the chance to meet 50 other patient activists from around the U.S. on a quixotic quest to safeguard the health care system. Most of us, like me, have suffered severe medical injuries in their families. The Institute for Healthcare Improvement selected us in a competitive process, convened us during their National Forum in Orlando, and lavished us with VIP-level care, through the generosity of Cari Oliver and Bill Thatcher of Cautious Patient Foundation, and Paul Levy of Beth Israel Deaconess Medical Center, among others.

> *"Kidney donors have a normal life span, a health status that is similar to that of the general population, and an excellent quality of life."*

Abraham, as described in the Book of Genesis, had faith so strong that he was willing to sacrifice his son Isaac. The Lord, as the story goes, spared Isaac. Many of my fellow activists have lost a son, daughter, husband, wife, father, mother. We are transmuting our anguish and our love into a passion for making health care safer and more effective and caring. My colleagues and friends in the emerging coalition of patient activists are living for others.

ALAN LEVINE'S STORY: THEY REFUSED TO RELEASE THE RESULTS

When my mother died in December 1998 at a Florida hospital, I asked a Medicare Quality Improvement Organization to review her death. I already had a copy of her medical record, and it appeared she received too high a dosage of an asthma medication. When the Florida Medicare Quality Improvement Organization refused to release the results of their review of my complaint, Public Citizen Litigation Group agreed to sue the Department of Health & Human Services on my behalf. At the time of the complaint, Quality Improvement Organizations operated under HHS policy that prohibited disclosure of information to beneficiaries. A January 2, 2001, New York Times news story on my lawsuit noted the following: "Tens of thousands of Medicare patients file complaints each year about the quality of care they receive from doctors and hospitals. But in many cases, patients get no useful information because doctors can veto the release of assessments of their performance... The new policy came in response to a lawsuit against the government by the son of a Medicare patient...The plaintiff [was] Alan Levine..." A July 16, 2001, letter from Amanda Frost, my attorney at Public Citizen, stated: "Enclosed is the opinion stating that the government must inform beneficiaries (or their representatives) of the results of investigations into beneficiary complaint. You should feel proud of your role in this case. Thousands of people will benefit as a result of your decision to stand up to the government and fight its policy of hiding medical errors."

I currently volunteer at Public Citizen Health Research Group where, for example, I have worked with an advocacy coalition on medical resident work hours. I also volunteer for Consumers Advancing Patient Safety (CAPS), where I chair their Advocacy and Policy Committee, and represent CAPS on the National Quality Forum Consumer Council (where I serve on the National Quality Forum's Patient Safety Steering Committee). I also volunteer for the Consumers Union "Safe Patient Project."

ARMANDO NAHUM'S STORY: THREE DIFFERENT TIMES

In 2006, my own family was infected with hospital-acquired infections three different times in three different hospitals in three different states within 10 months. Our son Josh, 27, died from his infection after it rendered him a permanent ventilator-dependent quadriplegic. Immediately afterwards, my wife Victoria and I co-founded Safe Care Campaign to educate the public and caregivers regarding best practices and how to prevent infections.

In 2007, our organization co-produced with APIC (Association for Professionals in Infection Control and Epidemiology Inc.) and the Centers for Disease Control (CDC) a five-minute video for use in-hospital called "Hand Hygiene Saves Lives." It is the medical counterpart of the airline passenger safety video required by the FAA (Federal Aviation Administration) at the beginning of every flight in the U.S. and was created to be shown to patients and their families upon admission to a hospital. The video educates as well as encourages patients to ask caregivers to wash or sanitize their hands before touching them. Thousands of acute care facilities across the country are using the video, changing the culture of "just take care of me" to one of shared responsibility and proactivity.

PATTY SKOLNIK'S STORY: THROUGH CAR FAX

Our son Michael is our hero and I will try to briefly explain his horrific experience of being in hospitals for 27 months. This was our tragedy. He was 22 years old and beginning nursing school when it happened. Imagine a scenario when your trust is broken at the ultimate plane of dependence and vulnerability. Imagine watching your child play victim for almost three years to a broken medical system. Michael had unnecessary brain surgery which caused him to be a severely disabled 6'4" infant. He could not move, eat, speak, and was 50 percent blind. He lived with horrific pain and was psychotic – these were the lasting outcomes. He had a g-tube, j-tube, super pubic tube, trach...27 medications ground with a mortar and pestle each day. The issues in the hospitals over that amount of time are too innumerable to list. Every complication possible occurred over and over again. Michael came home to our own ICU the last six months of his life until, on June 4, 2004, at 5:35 p.m., he mouthed the words "I love you" and took his last breath. He had just turned 25.

You can suffer a great loss, but you have a choice as to how to handle it. Anger and grief have a place, but taking that and transforming it

> into a solution is the best healer for everyone. I left corporate America to start CPS (Citizens for Patient Safety) to pursue the mission of educating ourselves, medical professionals and other generations to take action to minimize medical errors by having safe systems and quality care.
>
> Due to the terror we experienced I would fight for no more secrecy. On May 24, 2007, Governor Bill Ritter signed into law The Michael Skolnik Medical Transparency Act. On June 10, 2010, Governor Ritter signed into law the Michael Skolnik Expansion Act of 2010. We again had the support of all. All medical professionals licensed by DORA (the [Colorado] Department of Regulatory Agencies) will have a public profile showing the good, the bad, and sometimes the ugly, so consumers can make informed decisions about who is managing their health care. In a time when you can find out about a car you want to purchase through Car Fax we thought it time that consumers be able to have "Medical Professionals Fax."

Alan, Armando and Patty are focusing their life work on advocacy. Others have been able to make a great contribution at the end of their lives. A compelling example comes from the life and death of Randy Pausch. A professor at Carnegie Mellon University, Pausch was diagnosed with pancreatic cancer, and was invited to give a last lecture. It is now widely available.

> After I gave my lecture, I expected to go home and quietly spend time with my family. I never imagined that my talk would be viewed online by millions worldwide. The response has overwhelmed and moved me.

"When I encourage healthcare consumers to empower themselves, I'm describing something very different than girding yourself with the right armor for fighting battles with the adversaries, the practitioners."

> Thousands of people have written to me about their life lessons. I've also been buoyed by former students who've told me how my teaching made a difference to them. There's no greater gift for a teacher.
>
> I've used my unexpected fame to advocate for pancreatic cancer research. I testified before Congress to seek funding for my disease, which

is considered the deadliest of cancers. I am honored that my lecture will live on and that people have found it beneficial. Honestly, though, the talk was for my kids, and it gives me comfort to know that they will one day watch it.[1]

✚ **Communicate your most essential messages before it's too late.**

Randy was an empowered patient. When I encourage health care consumers to empower themselves, I'm describing something very different than girding yourself with the right armor for fighting battles with the adversaries, the practitioners. Rather, I'd like you to be able to speak powerfully for yourself, to achieve health in the fullest sense, however you might define that. Not just to be cured from disease, but to live as fully as you can, while you can. That means partnering with your doctors and nurses and friends. Randy wanted to leave a legacy for his young children and to equip them with at least some of the wisdom he had acquired. He found a way to do so that long outlasted him. Even better, he found a way to help a large number of people outside his family who may find themselves in similar situations. That's what makes him, Art Buchwald, Helen Haskell, Sorrel King, John James, Andy Levine, Patty Skolnik, Armando Nahum and our colleagues powerful and heroic patient advocates.

Christopher Field's contribution was less vocal but widely helpful, too. He was a history buff and a Godzilla fan. The 16-year-old youth suffered since birth from scoliosis and an unidentified condition that left his muscles weak. But he led a largely unimpaired life, using a wheelchair only for long walks.

At an appointment in the summer of 2005, doctors noted that his spinal scoliosis had worsened and suggested immediate surgery to save his internal organs. Nine days after the 14-hour surgery, Christopher developed pneumonia, and his breathing grew labored. He was brought to the ICU. He suffered a fatal blood clot in his lungs (a "pulmonary embolism").

His mother decided to donate his organs to needy patients, setting in motion a ripple effect of tissue donations that have reached as far as Portugal. Two people now can see – with his corneas. His bones have been used to prepare 39 bone grafts, with two transplanted already. Doctors have used his heart tissue to repair a defect in a young Massachusetts boy's heart. The New England Organ Bank counts almost 50 people who will ultimately benefit from Christopher's tissue donation.[2]

✚ **Carry an organ donor card in your wallet or purse.**

You don't have to die to be an organ donor. In 1967, doctors had asked Anthony Thein to donate one of his kidneys to help his brother. He did so, even though at that time, doctors didn't know whether living with a single kidney would harm his own health in the long run. It didn't. More than 40 years later, Anthony is now in his 70s and says he hasn't encountered any problems as a result. He regards the long scar across his belly with pride. Nowadays, donors' scars are much smaller. He regards his as "a badge of honor."[3]

A large study in the prestigious *New England Journal of Medicine*[4] finds that Anthony's experience was typical. The authors conclude, "Kidney donors have a normal life span, a health status that is similar to that of the general population, and an excellent quality of life; they do not have an excessive risk of ESRD [end stage renal disease]. The majority of donors in our study had a preserved GFR [glomerular filtration rate, i.e., the flow rate of filtering by the kidneys], and their rates of albuminuria [poor filtering out of a common protein from the urine] and hypertension [high blood pressure] were similar to those of matched controls."

Smaller gifts can help too, sometimes in surprising ways. As many political lobbyists know, some gifts benefit the giver, not just the recipient. This can be true in the public health domain as well, in a much more genuine way, as I learned from my primary care doctor. I was considering becoming a regular donor of blood platelets through apheresis, and was concerned about its long-term effects. He explained that my body would promptly replace the platelets, which could, if anything, have a stimulative effect on my own health. This may occur because the body replaces the older, donated platelets with new ones. Anyway, each platelet of a healthy person only lasts a week or so, and an adult of average weight has almost a trillion of them, plenty to spare. And I feel fine. Smug, even, to learn that my platelets go to people with leukemia or AIDS.[5]

So every three months or so I sit in a warmed Barcalounger kind of chair, wearing a blanket, attended closely by pert, funny nurses while I watch a movie I've brought. Afterward, they let me eat as many cookies as I want, though I don't need to. On the way out, I enter a raffle for free Red Sox tickets. I leave, feeling fine, and feeling virtuous. There are worse ways to spend two hours.

✚ **Donate blood.**

Having a strong purpose in life itself lengthens a person's life. It may be that living for others, as described here, or dedicating yourself to some similarly, hopelessly idealistic goal, will make you healthier, as well as those you care most about.

---

1. Randy Pausch, "The Lessons I'm Leaving Behind," Parade Magazine, April 6, 2008, pages 6-7.
2. Sarah Schweitzer, "Through tissue donation, a dear life goes on," Boston Globe, Jan. 1, 2008, pages B1 and B3.
3. Nathan Seppa, "Donating a Kidney Doesn't Hurt Long-Term Health," Science News, Jan. 28, 2009.
4. Hassan N. Ibrahim, Robert Foley, LiPing Tan, Tyson Rogers, Robert Bailey, Hongfei Guo, Cynthia Gross, and Arthur Matas, "Long-Term Consequences of Kidney Donation,"
N Engl J Med 2009; 360:459-469. Technical terms are explained via Wikipedia.org.
5. Background information from www.chp.edu/CHP/P02315 and Wikipedia.

CHAPTER TWELVE

Finding and Working with a Professional Patient Advocate

The decision to hire a professional advocate, or use an amateur, will be a difficult one because you'll be under stress, when it's hard to think clearly, and it may be hard to pinpoint and articulate what you need. You may never have had a health crisis that required a patient advocate. You'll need to consider whether to use a professional, and if so, how to find one. Then you'll need to know how to hire one. You'll need to know what kind of help to expect.

Because this will be such a new decision for most consumers, this chapter first shows how professional advocates have helped in a variety of situations, and then provides a menu of the kinds of tasks professional advocates perform, so you can decide what services you need. Guidelines for finding and hiring a professional advocate, or an amateur, follow that.

ADVOCATES' STORIES

In December 2010, when the Institute for Healthcare Improvement assembled the most fervent patient activists for a "Leadership Summit" to explore future roles for patient advocacy, as a fellow participant, I asked several of them to describe the most critical thing that patient advocates can do for an individual client. Together, their responses below paint a picture of what professional patient advocates can and should do for their clients.

> *"You'll need to consider whether to use a professional, and if so, how to find one. Then you'll need to know how to hire one."*

THAT FEAR WAS QUICKLY DISPELLED: ALAN LEVINE'S STORY

I recently hired a patient advocate (about $100 per hour) for my brother in Phoenix who was told he needed surgery to remove a cyst on his pancreas.

My brother used the patient advocate (who was a nurse) to accompany him to office visits for the many physicians he needed to see. The patient advocate researched the condition, the physicians, options for a second opinion, collected all his medical records (my brother signed a HIPPA waiver for the nurse's access), and stayed with my brother in the hospital.

It was expensive but worth every penny. The nurse advocate helped the communication amongst physicians, caught several communication problems in the hospital (including an infectious disease consult that was ordered but never followed up on), and asked questions of the physicians that only an informed person would know to ask.

Initially there was some resistance on the part of some of the doctors but ultimately they appreciated the "help." Also, my brother was somewhat apprehensive for fear that his doctors would not appreciate the intrusion. That fear was quickly dispelled as the nurse advocate became a valuable asset.

There was one incident at the hospital involving a supervisory nurse who did not like the nurse advocate asking questions and requesting certain things. That conflict was ultimately cleared up.

Alan Levine is a pro bono health care activist and advocate based in Washington, D.C.

AS DID THEIR PRE-OP INSTRUCTIONS: CARL FLATLEY'S STORY

I just had four back surgeries in the last two years. The fourth surgery solved the problem and I was told by the two operating surgeons that the first three surgeries were a waste of time! My insurance companies were billed between $400,000 and $500,000 for the procedures associated with the first three. Before all the surgeries I expressed concern about infection and sepsis [blood poisoning, a whole-body inflammatory state with a known or suspected bacterial infection]. Their attitudes changed as did the pre-op instructions!

Professional advocates should get multiple professional opinions and interview the patients that have had the procedure from that doctor. Empower patients to speak up. They do not have to be completely knowledgeable about the procedures, but they need to express concern about the outcome. If the doctor's mantra is first "do no harm," then the patient's should be "do not hurt me."

Carl Flatley, DDS, is the founder and chairman of the Sepsis Alliance, headquartered in Tampa, Fla.

THEY WANTED TO CHECK THE BINDER: JULIA HALLISY'S STORY

When my late daughter, Katherine Hallisy, was two years old she was diagnosed with a recurrence of cancer that required 36 rounds of chemotherapy. I was immediately faced with challenging responsibilities, such as learning to maintain and flush a central line at home, dressing changes, blood draws and managing a sometimes overwhelming amount of paperwork and other critical information.

I quickly realized that I needed a system to keep track of the chemotherapy protocol, blood test results, medications and symptoms. I assembled a binder with dividers and brought it to appointments and hospital visits. At first, our oncologist and the hospital staff seemed a bit uneasy about the binder but they soon realized what a valuable tool it was. I asked the nurses for copies of the medication administration records and blood test reports and I had the written report from every spinal tap, X-ray and scan. Soon, the doctors and nurses began to come into the room because they wanted to "check the binder" for a piece of vital information. The staff began to see the value in having someone close to the patient keep track of important details.

My binder was an early version of what is called a "Patient Journal" today. Our organization, The Empowered Patient Coalition, has a free patient journal available on our website at www.empoweredpatientcoalition.org/publications. Both patients and their advocates will benefit from keeping a record of all providers, medications and treatments. Patients who are involved in their treatment and have the assistance of an advocate will not only experience better outcomes, they will undoubtedly improve both health care safety and quality.

Julia Hallisy, DDS, is the president of the Empowered Patient Coalition, based in San Francisco.

TO SEE THEIR ROLE DIFFERENTLY: LORI NERBONNE'S STORY

After losing my mother to multiple lapses in care and failure to rescue, our family did our own form of "root cause analysis" and figured out that our mother's outcome may have taken a different course if we had felt more knowledgeable and empowered to raise the right questions assertively before and after her surgery, to follow/listen to our instincts, and to never back down until resolution. Although we understood fully that providers are the trained professionals in providing care, we also came to realize that partnering in our loved one's care is critical for improving outcomes. Patient advocates can build that bridge.

The most critical way that an advocate can help...in general [is] helping them to take the time to figure out what their personal needs are and then to communicate those needs clearly before and during a medical encounter. As an advocate, I ask, What is your agenda? What do you want out of this medical appointment or hospitalization? What do you want to gain out of raising your fears and concerns to the nurse? This helps them to see their role differently and from that we can often build a list of questions or input. It helps them to "extract" what they need from their provider.

Lori Nerbonne is the head of New Hampshire Patient Voices.

> *"There's a real gap between what doctors are saying and what patients are saying. I saw that kind of communication breakdown in all sorts of ways."*

THEY MIGHT'VE ATTENDED TO THAT: TANYA LORD'S STORY

My son had his tonsils taken out. He was very sick, so we brought him to the ER in Philadelphia, since he'd been throwing up and was very dehydrated. The doctors were treating him for dehydration, but not as a post-op patient. It seemed they were taking care of him appropriately, but later he hemorrhaged from the surgical site and died at home five hours after being discharged. I knew his dehydration was important, but I couldn't get the doctors to consider that there was something else wrong. A professional patient advocate could've gotten them to. If the advocate could have thrown in that little point, from their medical training or some other knowledge, they could have suggested trying something different. The doctors might have attended to that, if so.

A professional patient advocate can act as a translator between the family and the medical system. There's a real gap between what doctors are saying and what patients are saying. I saw that kind of communication breakdown in all sorts of ways.

Tanya Lord, who lives in Nashua, N.H., is studying in a doctoral program in patient safety at the University of Massachusetts Medical School.

A STARK AWAKENING: KERRY O'CONNELL'S STORY

I had a stark awakening back in 2005. I had a letter war going with the hospital on why I was responsible for paying over $80,000 in infection treatment costs. I walked into the risk manager's office one day to inquire about the status of my latest letter. She claimed they were not responsible for my infection as they did nothing wrong. I asked her if I had to sue them to get them to care. She responded, "Go ahead and sue us; you will never prove how that bacteria got into your arm." Obviously they don't care.

It is really good to have an observant advocate with an exceptional memory to witness the quality of care. Patients are too impaired by drugs, pain and anesthesia to really understand what is happening. Professional advocates can help by digging the truth about complication risks out of the providers, asking the really hard questions. Doctors never give you the whole story voluntarily.

Kerry O'Connell is the past chairman of the Colorado Health Facility Acquired Infection Reporting Committee, and is based in Conifer, Colo.

IT HAD ONLY BEEN HIS SECOND: PATTY SKOLNIK'S STORY

We didn't know what we didn't know and we "trusted" without question what the neurosurgeon said about the need to operate promptly on my son. The doctor claimed to have performed many such surgeries, but he later admitted in a legal deposition that Michael's procedure had only been his second.

An advocate can be the set of eyes and ears that the patient or close family member does not have at the time of making a critical decision. There must be shared decision making with informed consent in order to make the correct decision, one that could mean life or death as in Michael's case.

Patty Skolnik is the founder of Citizens for Patient Safety, based in Denver.

JUST LIKE HER BABY: MARY ELLEN MANNIX'S STORY

Recently, I helped a mom through a near-miss medical error at a leading pediatric hospital. Informing her of the resources available to her, how to access them, and remaining available to her helped her remain calm and focused to get the right care for her baby boy. I am happy to say he is home today and healing beautifully. Had I (or another advocate with insight) not been there, she said she never would have known where to turn and her son would be dead. For parents, the most critical role an advocate can play is to inform/educate/support the parent (who is the pediatric patient's advocate). Parents of sick children need support from an objective third party.

My husband and I did not have any of that when James was hospitalized. I had no idea who and what to ask. There was so much that was not afforded us at such a tender time. If we had what this mom had from me, James might be here. Just like her baby is now.

Mary Ellen Mannix is the founder and president of the STB Project and is the author of *Split the Baby*. She is based in Wayne, Pa.

OVERWHELMED IN A FOREIGN SYSTEM

The most powerful thing we can help patients and families understand is that they can do this! It's someone standing next to you, reminding you that you have strengths, no matter how small, to build on. When we feel overwhelmed in a foreign system, it's easy to lose sight of the fact that we do have some skills we can draw upon to manage our situation.

Libby Hoy is the founder of Patient & Family Centered Care Partners, an organization that strives to build partnerships between providers and their patients and families, in Long Beach, Calif.

SHE WAS NOT AN EASY PATIENT: BILL THATCHER'S STORY

My repeated participation in my mother's emergency room and hospital encounters as my mother neared the end of her life in her 80s showed missed medications, over-medications, competing medications from different doctors and miscommunications between my mother and the floor staff at the hospital. My mother was not an easy patient. Sometimes I thought she was the poster child for the "difficult patient" so I spent a good deal of time shmoozing the medical staff, smiling and acknowledging their individual "sainthood." Nonetheless, my mother deserved good care and I worked to ensure that she wasn't neglected just because she was who she was – difficult.

The most critical way that a professional patient advocate can help an individual client is by ensuring there is someone with the patient advocating for the patient 24/7, if they are in the hospital or whenever they come into contact with medical professionals. A close corollary to being present with the patient is ensuring that the patient and their advocate know their "rights" both generally to health care and specifically to the part of the health care industry in which they are engaged.

Bill Thatcher is the executive director of the Cautious Patient Foundation, based in Houston.

These stories hint at the range of services that patient advocates provide. A more explicit list appears below. The list focuses on the medical and navigational services described in this book; advocates also provide billing, insurance and legal services.

A MENU OF PATIENT ADVOCACY SERVICES

Before the doctor visit

- Address and ease your concerns

- Identify the key reason for the visit

- Help choose a doctor

- Interview past patients of that doctor

- Research the illness/condition
- Research treatment alternatives
- Prepare questions and convey to doctor
- Prepare a summary and convey to doctor
- Prepare the medication list and convey to doctor
- Empower patient, e.g., by rehearsing
- Collect relevant records, e.g., test results and previous progress notes
- Explain what will happen during the visit
- Help you learn about your condition
- Assemble a Personal Health Record

During the doctor visit

- Bring medications, vitamins and supplements from home
- Accompany the patient
- Record what is said, i.e., providers, treatments, follow-up instructions
- Verify clear understanding of self-care
- Ask what other diagnoses are likely
- Ensure the doctor and patient communicate clearly

After the doctor visit

- Get second or third opinions
- Help you learn about alternatives
- Explain to relatives
- Set up a reminder system to encourage you to perform the self-care the doctor suggested

- Check for drug-drug interactions
- Look into complementary/alternative treatment
- Gather and work through decision aids

Before the hospital procedure or stay

- Choose a hospital
- Choose a surgeon
- Ascertain wishes if patient can't speak
- Ensure an informed decision is made, clarifying risks and benefits
- Assemble music, clothes, etc.
- Ensure rights are known
- Explain what will happen in the hospital
- Ensure doctors have the information they need
- Clarify the patient's goals, needs and desires

During the hospital procedure or stay

- Empower the patient to speak up
- Verify that lab and diagnostic tests occur and results pertain to the right patient
- Mark the correct side of the body for surgery
- Compile hospital journal of care
- Verify medications are correct
- Obtain a care map for the condition
- Verify prophylactic antibiotics
- Learn and offer input to the discharge plan

- Communicate to other family members
- Track progress on the care plan
- Arrange multidisciplinary team meeting if needed
- Translate medical language
- Convey patient's concerns to medical team
- Verify that the treatment plan is being carried out
- Set up network of helpers after discharge
- Stay in the hospital
- Ensure follow-up on tests
- Witness the quality of care
- Nudge staff to wash their hands
- Provide emotional support
- Act promptly to minimize the harm of an error if one occurs
- Write clear terms of informed consent
- Discuss alternatives to ICU treatment with the patient or family

After leaving the hospital

- Fill in gaps in the discharge plan
- Ensure follow-up appointment is arranged
- Ensure self-care instructions are known
- Coordinate network of helpers
- Communicate to family members
- Take the patient home
- Find friendly support groups

- Arrange telemonitoring or reminders if needed
- Look into complementary/alternative treatments
- Follow up on substandard care if needed

A family member or friend may be able to help you, in lieu of a professional advocate. To ascertain if that's possible, first check off the types of services you'd like from the menu above. Then ask your family member or friend these questions:

CHECKLIST IN CONSIDERING YOUR FAMILY MEMBER OR FRIEND AS YOUR ADVOCATE

❐ Do you feel comfortable and knowledgeable in this situation?

❐ Do you have experience at this?

❐ This is a high-pressure situation, and I'd need you to be cordial with the doctors and nurses. How would you talk to them if you think they've made a mistake? Do you usually feel comfortable in sticking up for yourself in situations like that? Can you tell me how you handled a situation like that?

❐ If I'm in pain, or really in discomfort, would you expect to get upset, or would you be calm?

❐ Can you be there the whole time, 24/7?

❐ If I'm not getting good care, how would you know? Whom would you tell, and how?

I've checked off the things I want you to do for me on the menu above. Which of those do you feel comfortable in doing?

FINDING A PROFESSIONAL PATIENT ADVOCATE

- If you or they are not fully comfortable in their serving as a patient advocate, you should look for a professional.

- Since you probably don't know one, you can either ask well-connected nurses, doctors or health care professionals, or look in a network. Two growing networks of patient advocates are: the Professional Patient Advocate Institute (contact: cbrault@accessintel.com), and the AdvoConnection network (contact: Trisha Torrey, mail@diagknowsis.org).

- If you're already in the hospital, without an advocate, you can look for an advocate who is employed by the hospital. If so, you should test their responsiveness early on, before any crisis. Since they're paid by the hospital, they may not represent you as assertively as you might want.

HIRING A PROFESSIONAL PATIENT ADVOCATE

- Ask them to describe similar situations to this one, and ask how they helped.

- Ask for a written statement of the services they'll provide, along with what they expect from you, and their rate of pay.

- Ask for their references, and talk to them about what surprised them.

CHAPTER THIRTEEN

Partners in the New Contract

H ere's my daydream of how empowerment and partnership look in practice.

A few days ago I got a warm, funny postcard from my doctor, reminding me of my upcoming appointment, asking me to email him my medication list, and inviting me to email him with any questions I'd like to discuss. In the card, he congratulates me on the progress I've made on my fitness plan, which he has monitored by email since my last physical exam. (He'd asked whether I preferred a letter, postcard or email for the reminder, and since I'm not concerned about confidentiality, I preferred the postcard.)

A day or so before the visit, I email him my medication list, which my pharmacy had emailed me. It includes the over-the-counter chondroitin and glucosamine that I take regularly. I also had emailed him the topics I'd like to discuss. Patients who prefer writing on paper fill out a corresponding form in the waiting room on the day of the visit. Either way, the information lands in my electronic health record for future reference.

When I arrive, the assistant hands me some patient education materials about the condition I've mentioned, and I read it during the short wait to see my doctor. I know I'll get an electronic copy from him after the visit. He hands me the paper pamphlets because he knows I prefer that in his office.

In the exam room, the nurse takes my weight, blood pressure and pulse, and I can promptly see from the graphs on her iPad how they compare with my past readings. The doctor runs through the questions I've submitted. He refers to the problem list in my electronic medical record and the note that the ENT specialist had emailed into it, which recommended surgery for a benign nasal polyp. My primary care doctor discusses the trade-offs of different options and supports my decision not to have surgery for now. He advises me on how to use an inhaler that can shrink the polyp, forestalling or delaying the need for surgery. He realizes from the pharmacy's medication list and refill history that I've been using the inhaler every other day instead of daily, and we discuss that.

By the end of the visit, we have discussed my fitness plan and my risk factors. At the end of the visit, he hands me some printed information about my condition and his suggestions, emailing me a copy. On my way out I schedule a date for my next appointment. By the time I get home, he or an assistant has emailed me the website addresses where I can learn the most accurate information about my condition. Because he knows I have had a lot of formal education, he also suggests I read a particular review article in the medical literature. For patients with limited English proficiency, he recommends other materials.

This reflects a new and different mindset by the patient and doctor. As Lori Nerbonne says, "We are just so conditioned to leave everything in the hand of the provider that patients benefit from an approach that 'turns the table' so it can be viewed as a partnership that they are in control of. Much like when we go to a banker, or lawyer, or even to make a big purchase like a car...we have an agenda, we prepare ahead, we ask lots of questions, we speak up, we don't let the 'provider' be in total control.[1]

Different groups are trying to state the new rules. In its influential report, *Crossing the Quality Chasm*, in 2001, the Institute of Medicine listed 10 simple rules for the 21st century healthcare system.[2] More recently, John James has reshaped these into a bill of rights for hospital patients. The most recent draft appears on the next page; an earlier draft appeared in his book.[3]

The emerging partnership between patients and doctors is best imagined as an arranged marriage between two very different people who are resolved to make it work, and long past the honeymoon, have become good friends. In that spirit, where each partner has their own issues to work on, these are the patient's responsibilities, in Dr. Gordon Schiffs's vision:

- Push for timely access.

- Accurately and thoroughly describe symptoms and share your hunches.

- Write and prioritize questions in advance.

- Recruit your family or professional advocate for support.

- Read about the condition and drugs.

- Follow up after your visits by doing what you've agreed to do, noting how that's working for you and tracking delayed test results.

- Learn the greatest risks to your own health and address them.

- Write wishes for the end of life.

- Respect the limits on providers' time and society's resources.

- Agreeing to disagree where needed.

- Help in building and maintaining trust and communication.

- Participate in patient organizations.[4]

Along with these responsibilities, we have rights. It's time for us to see, and declare, our interdependence as equal partners. Our Patients' Bill of Rights is being drafted now. Let's turn the page.

---

1. Nerbonne: Lori Nerbonne, email communication, Dec. 9, 2010.
2. Institute of Medicine, Crossing the Quality Chasm: A New Health System for the Twenty-First Century, Washington: National Academy Press, 2001.
3. John James, A Sea of Broken Hearts: Patient rights in a dangerous, profit-driven health care system, Bloomington, IN: Author House, 2007.
4. Expanded and adapted from Gordon Schiff, "Understanding and Preventing Diagnosis Errors," a presentation to the Massachusetts Coalition for the Prevention of Medical Errors, July 17, 2010, Burlington, Massachusetts.

AMERICAN HOSPITALIZED PATIENT'S BILL OF RIGHTS

Medical Records: Patients shall be offered their medical record daily and be shown how to make entries into their record and correct any misinformation. Medical records shall be electronic by the end of 2011.

Evidence-based Care: Diagnosis and treatment shall be according to federal healthcare guidelines or according to peer-reviewed guidelines published by expert organizations for the medical condition of the patient. If the physician determines that a deviation from guidelines is needed, then the patient must be told that her care should deviate from guidelines and given an explanation for the deviation.

Therapeutic Drugs: No patient shall be prescribed a medication for off-label purposes without being informed that the drug prescribed has not been approved by the FDA for the patient's medical condition. The rationale for prescribing the off-label drug and the risk associated with this must be revealed to the patient. The patient shall be told how to report adverse effects of any prescription drug to the FDA.

Physician Competency: Patients have the right to be told the competency status of their physician before they are treated. This status shall include completion of state mandated CME, board-certification status, maintenance of board certification, rehabilitation from drug abuse, and any other factors that bear on the physician's competency.

Costs: Patients shall know the ordinary costs of the diagnosis and treatment that they are going to receive before they agree to a diagnostic plan or treatment plan. Treatment found to be against guidelines without the patient's consent does not have to be paid for.

Adverse Events: If an unanticipated adverse event occurs during diagnosis or treatment, the patient has a right to a full accounting of what happened and how the hospital intends to prevent similar adverse events in the future. If the adverse event was caused by a medical error, then the patient has a right to just compensation. Falsification of medical records after an adverse event constitutes tampering with evidence.

Duty to Warn: Patients shall know the hospital's infection rate and morbidity and mortality associated with planned invasive procedures. The patient shall be warned of any lifestyle activity that threatens their health. They shall be given guidance on management of that activity.

Informed Consent: The patient shall give their informed consent for invasive procedures according to guidelines published by the American Medical Association in 1998. Fear shall never be used to elicit consent for invasive procedures. Invasion of another person's body without genuine informed consent is battery.

Feedback on Care: The patient has a right, even a duty, to provide feedback to an independent agency on the quality of care they received during hospitalization. This feedback shall be systematically captured and made available to the public.

Advocate Present: All hospitalized patients have the right to have one advocate present in their room at all times.

Selection of Pathologist: The survivor of a deceased patient who died as a result of an adverse event has the right to have an autopsy performed by the medical examiner.

Appendix

A coda to *Getting Your Best Health Care*, the following excerpts culled from the Patient Safety Blog reveal some poignant insights and some maddening inconsistencies of our modern day healthcare system. These entries – the author's favorite choices – provide a fitting exclamation point to this book that strives for an exclamatory revision of our health and that of our medical system.

MY DOG HAS A BETTER MEDICAL RECORD THAN YOU DO

My dog Jackson had a well-dog checkup recently with his veterinarian.

A month earlier, we had received a postcard reminding us that he needed certain vaccinations and was due for a yearly checkup. (Does your doctor's office remind you?) When I phoned the office to make an appointment, they asked me my last name, and looked up his record on the computer so they could verify for me which shots he would need, and what the purpose of the visit would be. (Would your doctor's office do that?) Knowing he'd need a fecal test, they suggested I bring in a (poop) sample, and gave the necessary instructions. They entered the information into their computer scheduling program.

At the visit, much of the equipment was not much better than that of a doctor's office: a stethoscope to listen to his heart, a thermometer to measure his body temperature, a digital scale built into the floor, a pair of highly trained hands and eyes for the physical exam.

At the end of the visit, the vet handed me an individualized, four-page, neatly formatted and typed summary of what he had found, for each bodily system, with his advice on diet, exercise, and hygiene, a thumbnail photo of Jackson, lab test results and their interpretation, and target dates and types of future vaccinations. (Does your doctor routinely do that?) At check-out, I also received a receipt and itemized bill, which clearly named on an 8.5 x 11 inch sheet each shot and service Jackson had received, and showed the name of the receptionist, phone number, and future vaccine and exam dates, to keep for our records. (Does your doctor do that?)

They even advised on the preferred flavor of the toothpaste for daily brushing: poultry. The care was Mmm-Mmmmmm good!

Advice for people searching for a doctor: Find a doctor who uses an Electronic Medical Record to educate patients and themselves about the care you need.

MIRACLE ON THE HUDSON: LESSONS FOR HOSPITALS

It seems miraculous that US Airways Flight 1549 from New York City landed without loss of life in the Hudson River. The Jewish Talmud says, "Expect miracles, but don't count on them." The airplane designers apparently relied on this in their design of key safety features which enabled a skilled airplane crew to land the plane safely. Seven of their life-saving practices reveal life-saving suggestions for hospitals.

1. Captain Chesley Sullenberger III remembered from his training that if a plane has to ditch, it should be done near a vessel. So he landed the plane near a boat that he saw on that stretch of the Hudson. Other boat captains saw the first boat captain head toward the plane, and they followed, rescuing the passengers promptly.

Lesson for hospitals: Train doctors and nurses on what to do in case of errors as rare as needing to ditch a plane in the water.

2. The plane's first officer, Jeffrey Skiles, was in control of the plane at take-off. But as soon as the plane ran into the flock of birds and both engines quit at about the same time, the more experienced Captain Sullenberger announced, "My aircraft," using the standard phrasing and protocol drilled into airline crews during training. "Your aircraft," Mr. Skiles responded. The airline industry explicitly trains pilots how to manage the change of command of the plane, and the appropriate terse ways to communicate that. This hand-off of authority was clear, immediate, and was automatically documented in the

black box recorder. Trainers also teach crew members to routinely "say back" oral orders to ensure they have been correctly understood.

Lesson for hospitals: Create ways to hand off responsibility for patients that are clear, immediate, efficient, reliable, and verified.

3. After Captain Sullenberger took command of the plane, he, First Officer Skiles, and the air traffic controller discussed returning to La Guardia Airport, but decided against it. The pilot didn't decide alone; the three people took time to have a brief discussion, even in the midst of their extremely urgent looming disaster. Airlines have long trained pilots to perform such "crew resource management" (often now called "crisis resource management" in healthcare).

Lesson for hospitals: Train your clinicians to quickly, promptly and routinely discuss critical options for treatment, while driving out subordinates' fear that a higher-ranking surgeon or doctor will punish them for speaking up.

4. A passenger in the exit row was able to correctly remove the emergency exit door because he had taken a minute at that time to "readthelaminatedsafetycardofinstructionsintheseatpocketinfrontofyou." The airline had taken the time to prepare instructions for this very rare event of a water landing and place them where they could be snatched and understood promptly.

Lesson for hospitals: Patients are your partners. Help them by placing a laminated card of instructions in patients' rooms on how and when to call a Rapid Response Team. (It's now a state law in Massachusetts, and perhaps other places, for hospitals to have Rapid Response Teams to reply promptly upon the unexpected sudden deterioration in a patient's condition.)

5. After Captain Sullenberger took command of the plane, he set his co-pilot to work at moving through a three-page checklist of procedures for restarting the plane's engines. Note that the detailed checklist had been developed well in advance precisely for this exceedingly rare event. It was in the cockpit, i.e., it was immediately accessible, and didn't require the co-pilot to have memorized the procedures.

In this case, the checklist wasn't helpful, since it was intended for planes in distress at much higher altitudes, which allows for more time to restart the engines.

Lesson for hospitals: Sometimes you'll get lucky, and the patient will live despite your lack of a checklist. But you should, of course, have checklists for handling the most common errors. Expect laws soon to require the checklists.

6. The plane's force at impact would determine how many would live or die. It was critical to slow the plane. The pilots had to lower the flaps (movable devices on the wing) to slow the plane. But the flaps run on hydraulic power, driven by the now-useless bird-stuffed engines. The Airbus A320 has a "ram air turbine," essentially a little propeller, that drops down into the wind automatically in certain conditions, and produces electricity to provide the energy that allowed the crew to lower the flaps. With this automatic backup at work, the crew was able to slow the plane enough to make what felt like a hard landing, rather than a crash.

Lesson for hospitals: You may have generators that come into automatic use when the electricity fails. Perform a Failure Mode Effects Analysis to identify the failures that are most common and life-threatening, and ascertain where you need other automatic backups.

7. The Army Corps of Engineers is now searching the Hudson River for an engine, which may provide evidence on whether the plane really hit the birds. In effect, the government is helping to determine the cause of the accident.

Lesson for hospitals: Outsiders may be willing to help you find the causes of accidents. Let them partner with you.

THAT'S WHEN I CAN DO THE RELATIONSHIPS: INNOVATIVE DENTIST-PATIENT RAPPORT

An interview with my wonderful dentist, Herb Dorris, DDS, of Cambridge, Mass.

Why do you have so many posters and cartoons on the ceiling?

At first, I put things on the wall. I asked a patient what they thought: "But the ceiling is where we spend most of our visit, looking up there." But that's daffy!, I thought. I went into a restaurant, saw the blue ceiling and stars, and I noticed that kind of thing at other restaurants too. Maybe in my practice it'll be considered classy, like in the restaurants!

Why do you hand patients your own home-made educational materials at the end of the visit?

A patient told me, "You have a lot of good ideas [during the visit] but I don't remember anything!"

So I developed a newsletter, that I write about two times a year [about oral health and wellness]. That's what I hand out to patients, basically as an expression of my own craving for health and sanity. Because there are little ripples – for example, if you smile at somebody, it could make their day; who knows how it will ripple out? It may make a big difference in somebody's life.

How'd you come to have patients listen to music they like during visits?

Early in my career, it just felt so good. I felt it would be an alternative to injections and all the stuff we do that's intrusive. I must have picked it up through a personal experience, and it resonated.

Why do you do your own cleanings? I'm sure you give up some money by doing that.

It just came. That's when I can do the relationships; I like that a lot. When people want to connect with me especially during check-ups, they share their feelings with me and me with them. I like that. If I share personal experiences, I feel good, and I get a lot out of it.

But when I do fixing, I don't talk much – restorations, crowns, bite balancing – the reconstructive, repair part of dentistry – I'm a different person, in my own world.

What are your favorite days?

Check-ups, because I like people to become healthy, and I can shmooze more with check-ups. It's fun.

My brother was seven years younger than me. He almost dropped out, because he had encephalitis. He felt abandoned, and almost died, but he came back. I had the same feeling of abandonment during my early years. Several years later, I thought, if I can help my brother to make it, that will be fine. That's an underlying feeling. I won't be truly healthy in this lifetime, but if I can help others to do that, that will be fine. That's delightful to me; my presence is worth it. That, and sharing love, will make my life worthwhile.

ACKNOWLEDGEMENTS

I would like to thank the activists, advocates, members of the Consumers Health Quality Council of Health Care for All, and others who helped make this book possible:

Rick Atkins
Mark Bleier
Linda Burgess
Kathleen Clark
Jim Conway
Celestine Cox
Hinda Farbstein
Sondra Farbstein
Carl Flatley
Julia Hallisy
John James
Lester Hartman
Helen Haskell
Libby Hoy
Sorrel King
Linda Klein
Alan Levine
Tanya Lord
Mary Ellen Mannix
Rich Moche
Armando Nahum
Lori Nerbonne
Kerry O'Connell
Dori Peleg
Elizabeth Pell
Keely Sayers
Patty Skolnik
Kim Slack
Bill Thatcher
Rick Treitman
Nicola Truppin
Deborah Wachenheim
Lee Weinstein
Su Yoon
Alec Ziss

ABOUT KEN FARBSTEIN

Ken Farbstein is the founder of Patient AdvoCare, a company that advises patient advocates on keeping their family members safe and healthy while receiving medical care. In addition, he is the managing principal of Melior Consulting Group, an advisory firm for hospitals and other providers.

Ken writes the Patient Safety Blog (www.patientsafetyblog.com) to share real-life healthcare stories.

. . .

ABOUT PPAI

The Professional Patient Advocate Institute is a member organization and a community aligned around the common cause of providing advocacy for consumers as they strive to secure their healthcare needs and cover their insurance and financial matters.

PPAI offers a certificate program that provides comprehensive education for current and future patient advocates.
www.patientadvocatetraining.com